STRENGTH TRAINING

STAYING FIT & FABULOUS

CRIS CAIVANO

FOREWORD BY MICHAEL GEORGE

ixia
PRESS

MINEOLA, NEW YORK

About the Author

Cris Caivano is an exercise/movement therapist, educator, and certified Qigong instructor. Originally a dancer, she taught jazz dance to adults while also choreographing and performing. She became so intrigued by the needs and potential of her adult students that she refocused her work, studying dance therapy in London and receiving an M.A. in dance education from Columbia University. She created and ran dance/movement therapy programs at two psychiatric hospitals in Sacramento, and now lives and works in New York City and Dutchess County, NY, where she has an exercise/movement therapy practice specializing in adults over 50, but working with all ages. www.criscaivano.com.

Caution

The exercises described in this book are not to be considered substitutes for medical advice or treatment. Be sure to have a thorough checkup before doing these or any exercises. If you have a health condition, I urge you to learn if there are precautions you need to take before beginning an exercise routine. Your doctor can advise you as to what accommodations, if any, you may need to make.

Acknowledgments

Thanks to all my students, who continue to teach me more each day. Thanks also to Cathy Loup and Zanne Stewart for their help and encouragement during the writing of this book, and to my wonderful agent, Judith Weber.

Dedication

This book is dedicated to my parents Meg and Rocco, who taught me how to love the simple things.

Bibliographical Note

This Ixia Press edition, first published in 2017, is an unabridged, slightly revised republication of the work originally published by MQ Publications Limited, New York, in 2005. Color photography from the original publication appears in black and white in this Dover edition.

Library of Congress Cataloging-in-Publication Data

Names: Caivano, D. Cristine, author.
Title: Strength training: staying fit and fabulous / D. Cristine Caivano ; Foreword by Michael George.
Description: Ixia Press edition. | Mineola, New York : Ixia Press, 2017. | Includes index. | "This Ixia Press edition, first published in 2017, is an unabridged republication of the work originally published by MQ Publications Limited, New York, in 2005. Color photography from the original publication appears in black and white in this Dover edition" — t.p. verso.
Identifiers: LCCN 2017024837| ISBN 9780486818887 (paperback) | ISBN 0486818888
Subjects: LCSH: Physical education and training. / Muscle strength. | BISAC: HEALTH & FITNESS / Exercise. | HEALTH & FITNESS / Healthy Living.
Classification: LCC GV711.5 .C35 2017 | DDC 613.7/0446—dc23
LC record available at https://lccn.loc.gov/2017024837

IXIA PRESS
An imprint of Dover Publications, Inc.

Manufactured in the United States by LSC Communications
81888801   2017
www.doverpublications.com

contents

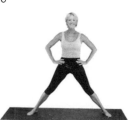

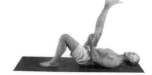

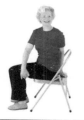

foreword by Michael George

Getting older has never been better for you. Today, most of us are living longer, staying fitter, and putting ourselves first. With the proper motivation, anything is possible. It doesn't matter how old or how fit you are—you can always integrate exercise into your lifestyle.

I grew up as a chubby kid with poor eating habits until my early teenage years, when I discovered sports and exercise. Once I incorporated consistent exercise into my daily life, the excess body fat dissipated and I became a much stronger and more confident person. But all of us, both young and old, need to look after our mental and physical health. The two are inextricably linked: Positive affirmation allows you to pursue a better body, and a better body can permanently lift your mood.

This fun and challenging book will help the older trainer "rediscover" his or her body, beginning with the basics: posture, breathing, and motivation. With constant reassurance and encouragement, Cristine Caivano introduces and explains exercises for the lower body, upper body, back, and abdominals. The entire body is given a thorough workout, and Cristine offers many variations designed for differing degrees of fitness. There is a chapter devoted to the special health concerns of the 50+ audience, as well as a series of carefully constructed programs for specific issues, such as the lower back.

Over the years, I have worked with many older clients, and I have to say that once they began a regular exercise program, each and every one of them experienced a better quality of life due to increased strength, stamina, and flexibility. Many of these clients also reduced their cholesterol levels, blood pressure, stress levels, and pain levels that were the result of structural problems or weakness.

I agree with Cristine's simple advice: Don't over-exert yourself, but exert yourself! You don't necessarily need to feel the burn to feel better. Gentle exercise is nothing to be afraid of, and you *will* reap dividends. It doesn't matter if your bones creak and your muscles feel stiff. If you participate in gentle, daily exercise, you will start to see a striking improvement in your mental and physical health. But why is this so important to the older adult? After the age of 50, we begin to slowly lose muscle and gain fat. Strength training in later life can slow down this process. It can also improve your flexibility and balance, helping you to avoid bad falls, guard against weak bones, relieve the symptoms of arthritis, and give you a stronger heart, a clearer mind, and a good night's sleep!

A healthy body means a healthy mind, and I hope that with the exercises in this book you too can find a happy equilibrium at a point in your life when you have the most time to enjoy it. Start training with this book and you'll never look back—I promise you. So start training and get stronger. You know you can do it!

About Michael George

Michael George is transforming the health and fitness industry with his innovative training philosophies and inspirational voice. He has become one of Hollywood's most sought after fitness experts and certified training consultants.

As an on-camera fitness personality, Michael demonstrates his non-traditional approach: a combination of health and fitness knowledge, motivational psychology, highly diversified athletic talent, and the mind/body connection. Michael has transformed some of Hollywood's most dynamic bodies, including those of actors Richard Dreyfuss, Meg Ryan, Christian Slater, Julianne Moore, Sela Ward, Miguel Ferrer, and James Spader.

the big picture

Most of us would agree it feels different to be 50 or 60 or 70 years old now than it did during our parents' lifetime. Medical advances and society's evolution have helped lead us to this point. Statistically, we will live longer than our ancestors. Some of us are beginning new careers and even new families at an age when our ancestors were sliding into peaceful retirement. Things have changed.

But one thing hasn't changed: No matter how young we may feel, or look, or act, we are still subject to the laws of nature. The human body and mind alter as they age. Some of these changes—wisdom, depth of character, self-knowledge—are wonderful. Others aren't so great, like the fact that, unless we stay physically active, we typically lose an average of 30 percent of our muscle mass by the age of about 70, and another 10 percent per decade after that. These are dramatic facts, but even more dramatic is your opportunity to avoid and even reverse these problems by making strength training an ongoing part of your life.

The MacArthur Foundation Study of Aging in America recently determined that even more than "choosing your parents wisely" (in other words, your genetic inheritance), three factors will influence the quality of your life as you grow older. They are: avoiding chronic disease, getting sufficient physical and mental activity, and maintaining social connectedness. A smart way to accomplish all of these goals is to begin by building your muscular strength. That way, you will have the energy, independence, confidence, and health to continue doing all the things that you enjoy and that promote an enjoyable life.

It is a widely held misconception that as we get older our bodies stop responding to exercise. This is totally false. Most of the time, we "lose" our strength and energy simply because we have stopped moving, playing, participating, trying. We give up. We don't use it, so we lose it. The sooner we reverse this trend, the more health capital we will accumulate, just like socking away money in a savings account. And the benefits will continue to accrue with the years. Just as we work to raise our children the right way as an investment in their future, so we must now invest in our future, by taking care of ourselves.

Let's face it—growing through life isn't easy. Yes, we can make amazing and empowering choices to assure our health and well-being, as far as anything in life can be assured. But we also need to have fun. We need to feel good as often as possible, and spread that good energy around. We need the strength to support ourselves and our loved ones during difficult times. Strength training is a great way to accomplishing all these things.

Cris Caivano

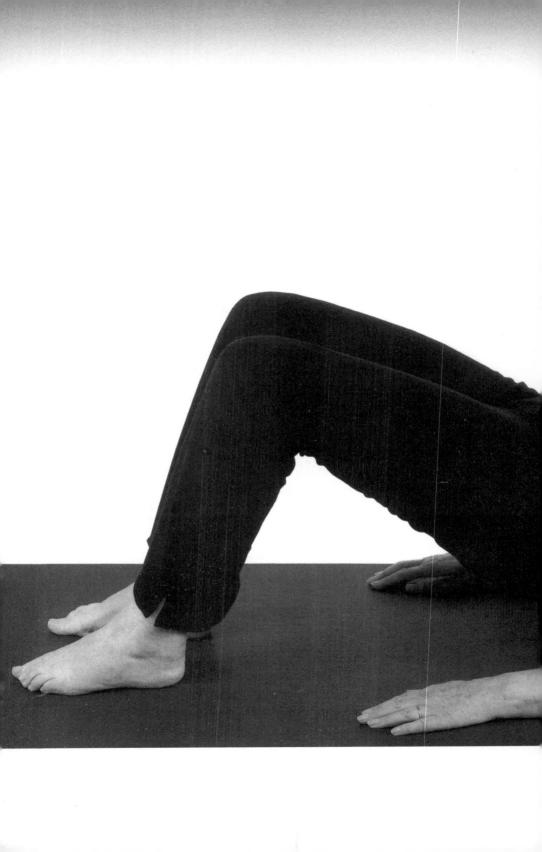

part 1 **getting started**

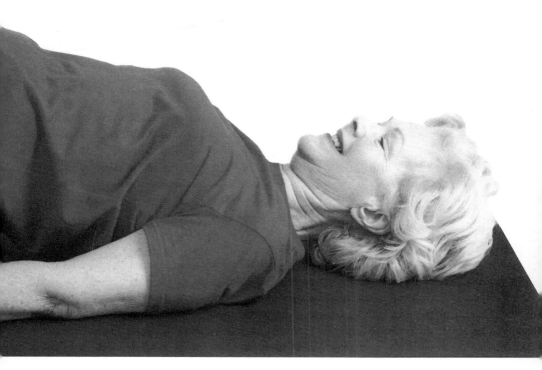

Why Strength Training is Important if You Are over 50

Scientists estimate that the average man will lose about 7 pounds (3.2 kg) of muscle each decade after age 25 if he doesn't do anything (such as strength training) to reverse this process, and the average woman will lose 5 pounds (2.3 kg) of muscle per decade after age 35. After menopause a woman's average muscle loss will occur at twice that rate, making her lose an average of a pound of muscle a year. That means a 60-year-old woman who doesn't do strengthening exercise will have lost over 10 pounds (4.5 kg) of muscle, even if her weight stays the same! This age-related loss of muscle is called "sarcopenia." Many of the characteristics we associate with aging—low energy, weakness, achy joints, and loss of movement confidence—are actually the side effects of decreased muscle mass.

Another unwelcome side effect of age-related muscle loss is "middle age spread." Muscles require lots of energy (calories) in order to maintain themselves and perform their job of moving and stabilizing the bones. If by becoming sedentary over the years you allow that age-related loss of muscle to occur, *and* you do not lessen your caloric intake proportionately, then you will get fat. It's just simple arithmetic: calories in, energy out—or fat on!

Can this loss of muscle be reversed? Absolutely! By committing to a strength-training program and sticking to it, you will rebuild the muscles that have disappeared, no matter how old or out of shape you are. Strong evidence from recent studies has shown that along with increased lean body mass, improved metabolic rate, and better weight management, the benefits of strength training include improved balance and coordination. You will be less susceptible to falls and other injuries, whether playing touch football or walking down a steep flight of stairs.

Strength training also helps prevent heart disease and adult-onset diabetes, and builds bone density in postmenopausal women and older men. It has even proven effective against depression. This disease preventive aspect is one of strength training's most underappreciated gifts.

But let's get to the fun stuff: Strength training will help you look and feel fabulous. Its effects are steady and cumulative; you will experience the immense pleasure of creating a new you, literally. This is quite empowering for us over-50s. You will, through the techniques in this book, learn how to grow your own beautiful, strong muscles, thus slowing the apparent and biological age of your body. As your muscles grow stronger you will notice a marked increase in your energy levels. Your self-confidence will increase and so will your independence.

Of course this is not the only thing you need to do to create such success; you must also be sure to eat properly, get enough rest, make cardiovascular training a daily occurrence (a 30-minute walk can get you started on that), and follow sensible rules of self-preservation, such as not smoking at all, or drinking too much. Strength training is a particularly good place to begin rebuilding your fitness, however, because it will make everything else you do so much easier!

Reassurance to the Out-of-Shape, Embarrassed, Intimidated, or Injured Exerciser

Did you know that encouraging research done in the past 10 years shows that even people in their 90s can increase their muscular strength in as few as *eight weeks*? Whatever your age, no matter how out of shape or inexperienced you are, you can markedly improve your strength. In fact, the more out of shape you are, the more dramatic your improvement will be.

This book will teach you what you need to pay attention to, in order to achieve results and avoid injury. I have made a point to include only time-tested, safe, and simple exercises. Throughout you will be reminded to "feel" your way through an exercise, to listen to your body, and to remember that *you* are the expert; if something doesn't feel right to you, don't do it. It's that simple. You are the boss and can choose how intensively to work. (Of course, the more consistent you are with your workouts, the faster you will achieve those satisfying results.) You will be surprised how quickly you begin to feel better once you start moving.

Women and Strength Building

Some women are concerned they will build unattractively bulky muscles from lifting weights. This won't happen, because women don't have enough male hormones circulating in their bodies to allow for such muscular growth. Your muscles will become more defined and shapely, but not necessarily much larger. In fact, your newly strengthened muscles will take up less space than fat tissue, so you will probably look slimmer as you get stronger.

One interesting fact we have always heard is that men have more upper body strength. That's because their upper body muscles and bones are larger than most women's to begin with. However, there is not an appreciable difference in the overall strength-building *potential* for men and women, once you take into account that difference in size. Women may have smaller bone structure and therefore smaller arm, shoulder, chest, and upper back muscles, but, contrary to popular belief, those smaller muscles can be trained to achieve big strength.

The ideas offered in this book apply to anyone. Just remember that age *is* relative. The concepts, techniques, and exercises described here will help an out-of-shape 25-year-old as much as a person three times that age.

below > Strength training will help you look and feel fabulous.

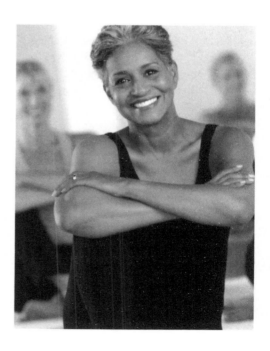

How to Use this Book

This book will teach you how to create your own strength-building workout. Only the essentials have been included. Before getting to the exercises, please read The Basics of Building Strength (pages 16–21). This section includes interesting, even surprising, information based on recent research, explaining how to accommodate the needs and quirks of your over-50-year-old body in order to get the best results from your workout. For instance, you will learn how correct alignment, coupled with strong core support, will enable you to do exercises that you may previously have found too difficult.

Two Foundational Exercises, the Squat (pages 37–41) and the Push-Up (pages 45–47), serve as an excellent starting point for your strength training. Both exercises work several different muscles at once; this allows you to make good use of your workout time as you strengthen and prepare your body for more focused exercises in Part 2: Getting More Specific.

The Props You Need

For some of these exercises, you will need two sets of weights. The smaller set will allow you to begin strengthening your muscles without working them to exhaustion, giving you the chance to learn correct form while also building stamina. The heavier set will provide a greater challenge once you are ready for it. In general, women who are healthy but unused to strength training might consider beginning with one pair of 3-pound (1.5 kg) weights and one pair of 5-pound (2.5 kg) weights. Men in the same situation should use a pair of 5-pound (2.5 kg) and a pair of 8-pound (4 kg) weights. Again, this

is an estimate. If you are very elderly, out of condition, or recovering from illness or injury, consider doing the exercises without using any weights at all until you feel stronger and more confident. At that point, begin with as heavy a weight as you can lift 10 times without fatigue (see also overload principle and repetitions, page 16).

Some exercises require a stability ball. It's important that the ball you use is the right size to provide adequate support and stability. To select the correct size, check that when seated on the ball, your knees are at about hip height, or slightly higher.

below > Choose your weights according to your level of fitness.

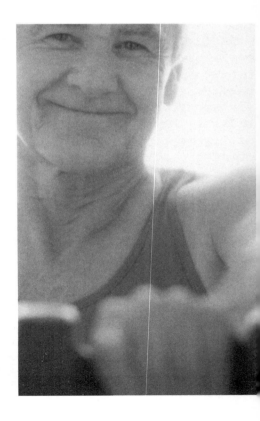

You may also want to work on an exercise mat. This keeps your feet from slipping and adds some cushioning for the lying-down positions and for bare feet. You can choose from special exercise mats or the thinner ones designed for yoga.

One more note: It's wise to wear sneakers when lifting weights. They help protect your feet and steady your balance.

Variations and Stretches

Many of the exercises include several variations so that you can work at your own pace. The Beginning Level exercises teach basic form and technique; do them first, for as long as you need, and return to them whenever you'd like to check up on your form. Be sure to follow your body's signals when deciding whether or not to try the more advanced variations. There's no rush! Whatever exercise is appropriately challenging to you is the one that will bring the best results.

Nearly every exercise is followed by a suggested stretch. That's because once you have worked a muscle enough to strengthen it, it will be warmed up and thus well prepared to stretch. By taking the time to stretch you also give your muscles a chance to rest before tackling the next strengthening exercise.

Planning a Personalized Workout

The structure of this book is, roughly, the outline of a good workout. Keep this in mind when you put together your own program. Try to work on your strength and flexibility at least twice, preferably three times a week, and allow one day's rest between all workouts. You may also want to look at the Programs (pages 138–151) for suggestions as to how you can organize the exercises to accomplish specific goals. Here are some general rules to help you organize your workout plan:

■ Always warm up first.
■ Work from larger muscles to smaller ones.
■ Work the muscles on the front of the body followed by the muscles on the opposite side.
■ Alternate between upper and lower body exercises.
■ Always work your abdominal muscles.
■ Don't neglect strengthening your back.
■ Stretch often and carefully.
■ Finish with a cool-down.

And just one last point to note: Our photographs don't lie. They show Tiffany and Greg, aged 56, and Tessa, aged 67.

The Main Muscles of the Body

You will find it easier to strengthen your muscles if you take a moment to study their shape, location, and relative size. By learning to visualize your muscles as you move, you will greatly increase the effectiveness of the exercises. Visualizing the muscles allows you to "tune in" with accuracy to what you are doing, enabling you to direct your efforts to where they will do the most good.

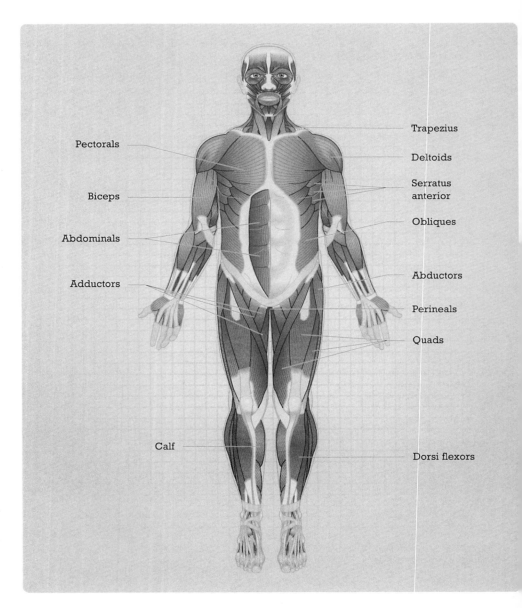

Pectorals

Biceps

Abdominals

Adductors

Calf

Trapezius

Deltoids

Serratus anterior

Obliques

Abductors

Perineals

Quads

Dorsi flexors

Look, for example, at the trapezius muscles. One of these muscles' "jobs" is to pull the shoulders down and back, thus contributing to good postural alignment. By knowing—and visualizing—their shape you will find it easier to enlist their help in exercises like the Scapular Squeeze on page 31.

At the beginning of each exercise section in this book, you will see a drawing of the muscles you will be using, highlighted in a box at the top of the page. This will help you understand where, exactly, you should be "feeling it" as you do the exercises that follow.

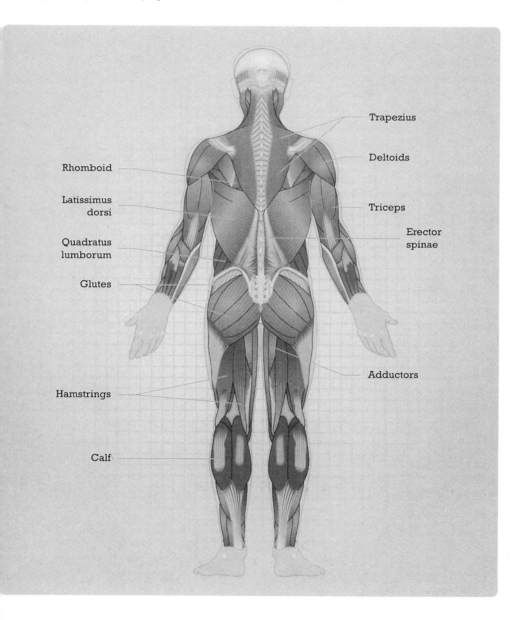

Trapezius

Deltoids

Rhomboid

Latissimus dorsi

Triceps

Quadratus lumborum

Erector spinae

Glutes

Adductors

Hamstrings

Calf

The Basics of Building Strength

Strength Training

To strengthen a muscle you need to push it slightly beyond its usual capacity, gradually increasing the intensity of this effort over time. This is what is known as the "overload principle."

When a muscle is challenged, by lifting a weight over and over again, for example, changes occur deep in its tissues. This sometimes leads to some soreness the next day. No studies have yet proven exactly why this happens. Some scientists believe that tiny, microscopic tears cause this minor soreness; others think it is a chemical response of some sort. Whatever its source, when you rest, your muscles repair themselves, healing in the form of stronger, more resilient muscle. That is why it is recommended that you do not work on strengthening the same muscle two days in a row. Generally, one day's rest between workouts is enough to allow that strengthening repair to occur. (You can strength-train daily: just alternate muscle groups from day to day.)

Your task, as an over-50 exerciser, is to challenge your muscles enough to get the benefits of the overload principle, but not so much that the normative, constructive stress turns into injury.

To apply the overload principle, use weights heavy enough that the muscle you are using becomes fatigued after about 10–15 repetitions, or "reps." If you can easily lift the weight for many more reps than that, then you need to increase the weight a bit at a time until you reach that 10–15 times limit. This applies no matter how much weight you are lifting.

If you are using a heavy enough weight, you will receive benefits from just one set.

Are you feeling strong and motivated? Then by all means, go for that second or third set. Your results will be even more impressive. Just be sure to rest between sets, either by doing a different exercise for one set, or by stretching.

In the beginning you may not be sure how hard to push yourself. This is when you should trust your perception. Your goal is to tire out the muscle, to use it more than it is accustomed to being used, in order to stimulate its growth. This will cause some mild discomfort, but should never cause any pain, especially not a jabbing or burning pain. Err on the conservative side, especially at the start. You may want to begin by doing the exercise without holding any weights at all if you are very out of shape.

If you cannot maintain correct alignment or form—for instance, if your back always arches up off the floor during an abdominal exercise—then leave that exercise for a while and return to one that you know you do correctly but that still offers a constructive challenge.

You should also monitor your breathing. Take a break, or slow down if you find yourself struggling for breath. You will always make better progress by working with your body, not against it.

And last but by no means least, don't be deceived into thinking that only painful, sweaty exercise will improve your strength. Of course there is always discomfort involved when we push ourselves beyond our current limits, but forget "going for the burn." You'll just get hurt. Indeed, the "no pain, no gain" slogan has been totally discredited by all sensible and well-trained exercise professionals.

Flexibility

Flexibility refers to the range of motion of the joints and limbs. If your muscles have grown stiff from lack of exercise, you won't be able to move freely. Adult muscles have lost about 15 percent of their moisture content, becoming stiff and unyielding. Stretching stimulates the production of muscle tissue lubricants, thus slowing down this gradual drying-out process.

As you stretch your muscles you will be surprised how quickly you start to feel better. Stretching helps to increase the circulation of oxygenated blood throughout your body. You will feel relaxed, revived, and may even be able to think a bit more clearly, as that oxygen reaches your brain.

As an over-50-year old, how you go about stretching is of great importance. Here are the facts to keep in mind.

❶ Warm Up: You should warm up for at least 10 minutes before stretching. Cold muscles will not stretch safely or well. Warming up will increase your circulation and also speed the transmission of nerve impulses to the muscles, preparing them to stretch and helping you avoid injury.

❷ The Stretch Reflex: The stretch reflex is like a conversation between the muscle that is stretching and the brain. If we didn't have this proprioceptive, protective mechanism, we would fling our limbs around beyond what is safe and cause extensive muscle damage. When the stretch begins, a signal travels from the muscle to the brain, saying something like "Whoa! We haven't done this in a while." The brain sends back an instantaneous command: "Don't move! Hold tight! Something unusual is going on down there and it might not be pretty!" The muscle

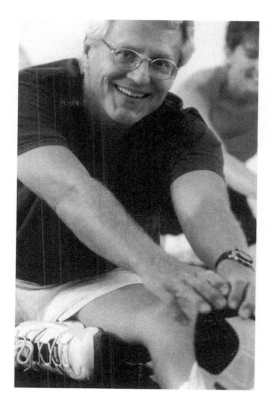

above > Stretching inhibits the gradual drying out of the muscles that is part of aging.

does as it is told by the brain; it stays contracted, perhaps even tightens further, to prevent this unfamiliar stretch from going too far and damaging the muscle fibers. It's kind of like playing tug-of-war with a strong puppy. The harder you tug, the more tightly the dog grabs the rope with its teeth.

After a few moments—generally speaking, at least 20 or 30 seconds—the brain recognizes that the muscle isn't in danger and gives the green light. The stretch reflex goes away and the muscle is free to begin to lengthen. (The moment is easy to identify, once you know to look for it.) To make a long story short—and a short muscle long—you cannot rush a stretch.

Alignment

Alignment refers to how your bones are stacked up in relationship to gravity, the force that draws our weight downward, toward the center of the earth. When your bones are properly aligned, they can support the weight of your muscles and internal organs. Your movements will be efficient and stress-free. Out of alignment? You are inviting trouble, especially when exercising, where poor alignment might lead to injury.

Good alignment can help you avoid aging prematurely. Think of it: What looks worse than sagging posture, a caved-in chest, that appearance of having been defeated by life 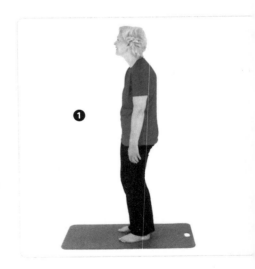?

Even worse than its effect on your appearance, poor posture is one of the most insidiously destructive things you can do to your body. Slouching compresses the lungs and other internal organs, impeding your breathing, circulation and digestion. It also places tremendous stress on the spine, its intervertebral discs, and supporting muscles. Just as we realign our car to avoid wear and tear on its various movable parts, so too correct postural alignment will help protect you from many aches, and injuries.

What, exactly, *is* good alignment? Try this:

You will need a mirror or maybe a partner to help you observe your postural habits. Stand in your usual way. Pretend you are on line at the post office, or any other scenario where you are not consciously focused on your posture.

Observe your body's profile. The center of your ear should be over the center of your shoulder. Drawing an imaginary line down from there, your shoulder should be above the center/side of your hip ❷. The

plumb line down from the hip should fall slightly behind the kneecap, then continue down to the knobby bone on the outside of your ankle ❸. This stacks the weight of the body parts one above the other, like children's blocks. Ear-above-shoulder-above-hip-above-ankle is the Basic Law of Alignment.

Still observing your profile, notice the three major curves of the spine: forward at the back of the neck, back over the ribs, then forward again at the back of the waist. These curves are your natural shock absorbers and are, indeed, built into the very structure of your 27 vertebrae. They allow the weight of the body to be transferred safely through the spine and pelvis, into the two legs and feet. Many people have the misconception that these curves are bad and try to stand in a ramrod-straight, soldierlike posture. This is a big mistake. Similarly, problems will occur if the curves are exaggerated. Anatomists call these healthy spinal curves "natural curves." When the three spinal curves are present but not exaggerated, it is called "neutral back."

Whenever you exercise, and especially before lifting weights, take a moment to observe the way your body is aligned. If your head is jutting forward, gently move it back, over the spine. Is your lower back swayed into an exaggerated arch? Then pull your abdominal muscles in and up, as if tucking them under your rib cage.

Learning to self-correct your alignment like this until it becomes an automatic habit, is without question one of the most important strengths you can develop.

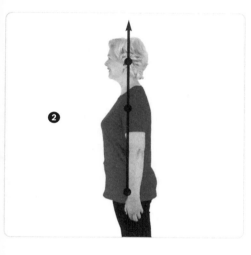

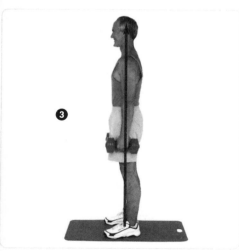

Breathing

When you are strength training, the manner in which you breathe is quite important. It can make everything you do a little easier, and much more pleasant.

Many exercise descriptions offer suggestions as to when to exhale and when to inhale. In general, it's helpful to exhale at the most challenging point of the exercise. For example, when you are doing a push-up, try to inhale as you lower your body, then exhale as you straighten your arms. It'll help give you that extra "oomph" that you need. If the breathing instructions offered here don't work for you, feel free to invent your own pattern as long as you *never, ever* hold your breath.

Breathing also has an important effect on your alignment. By exhaling thoroughly you draw the abdominals closer to the spine, creating stabilizing core support for your back. Make this a continually strengthening habit, whether you are exercising or just going for a stroll.

In general, be sure to take full advantage of every breath. Do you tighten your belly, breathing only into the small, upper regions of the lungs? If that is the case, you aren't receiving the fullest volume of breath possible. Be sure to relax your belly as you inhale, drawing the breath deep into the larger, lower lobes of the lungs. Then allow the belly to flatten inward on the exhale.

Last but not least, whenever you stretch, take slow, deep breaths. This sends an instant message to your parasympathetic nervous system, creating a state of relaxation. Your blood pressure will drop, your muscles will be better able to lengthen, and you will supply those newly flexible muscles with nourishing, strength-building oxygen.

Tuning In: Mindfulness

One of the most important skills you will acquire as you learn how to increase your strength is the ability to "tune in," to feel with accuracy the current state of your body. This tuning in, or mindfulness, requires honest and nonjudgmental self-observation, which, for many of us, is not an easy task! This is especially true if you are unhappy with the way your body feels, looks, or moves. You may be depressed by the changes that have occurred over the years, either to your mobility or your waistline. The last thing you may be willing to do is look closely at yourself. But by learning to tune in to your body, you will access truly amazing power to change the way you feel. You will gain control. Exercising will become a pleasure, not another chore to be dreaded.

Each exercise you do, indeed, each breath you take, can instantly transform your state of being if you take the time to observe, to feel, to tune in. This skill of refamiliarizing yourself with yourself will become easier the more you practice it. In time, tuning in will become completely automatic. It will feel as natural as noticing the smell of fresh coffee, or recognizing a friend's face in a crowd.

Mindful tuning in requires a mixture of focus and relaxation. Think of how you would pet a soft, cuddly young puppy. You would give the puppy your full attention, and you would soften your hands, so as to better feel the silkiness of the puppy's warm fur. If you approach your body, as achey and out of shape as it may feel, with the same gentle, relaxed focus, you will encourage profound improvements to occur.

Although at times you may feel stuck in a state of unfitness, know that your body is constantly changing and renewing itself.

Every moment thousands of cells are dying and are being replaced by new ones. Your environment is always changing, your moods, your strengths and vulnerabilities are in a constant state of flux. This is true even if you are 95 years old. It only makes sense to try and observe these daily changes with a fresh pair of eyes.

Refamiliarizing yourself with your body in a gentle and precise manner will help you to differentiate the discomfort that often accompanies new ways of moving—the "good pain"—from the "bad pain" of forcing your body to do something it is not yet ready for. That is why tuning in helps you avoid the injuries that can result from exercising in a careless or distracted manner. At the same time, by always moving with awareness and attention, you will possess the confidence to know when you are ready to take on a bigger challenge, such as lifting heavier weights, trying a more difficult variation, or balancing on one foot.

Throughout this book there are frequent reminders to observe the way your body is responding to each exercise. It matters that you can learn to relax your shoulders and sense the muscular support of your deep core. It matters that you know that by inhaling and exhaling in a mindful manner, you will protect your heart as well as build strength and flexibility more quickly and easily. It matters that you come to feel the influence that standing in good alignment has on your strength and energy. This tuned-in approach to building strength is very motivating, because it transforms exercising into a fascinating, rewarding experience. You may be surprised to find that you actually begin to look forward to your workouts, and I am sure that you will be delighted by your steady progress.

Motivation

Even the most committed athletes have days when they feel like not moving. If you find yourself immobilized by inertia or lack of enthusiasm, here are a few simple ways to nudge yourself into action.

Just get through the first 10 minutes. Get out your exercise mat. Lie down and do one stretch—just one—whatever feels good. Breathe. Take your time and give the stretch your full attention. Once you do that you'll want to do another. Then another. Before you know it, you're warmed up, in a better mood, and ready to do a full workout.

Weave exercise into your day. When you are feeling peppy do 10 or 15 minutes of an exercise you find challenging. Later in the day do some seated stretches. Take a quick, 15-minute walk two or three times a day, instead of struggling to find 45 minutes of uninterrupted time. Do Heel Raises while waiting for the kettle to boil.

Try making daily exercise appointments with yourself. "Not enough time" is a common reason to avoid exercising. Schedule it in, before other events distract you or interfere. This will help you get into the habit of working out regularly.

Work out with a buddy. Team up with a friend, and commit to exercising together. Even if you don't feel like working out, you won't want to let down a friend, and that may be all the motivation you need.

Anticipate the "chain effect". There are times, for example, especially when you first start exercising, when you may feel discouraged by an apparent lack of progress. Be patient—the "chain effect" is gathering itself. At some point, the subtle improvements that are occurring in your body should accumulate and enhance each other. You may then experience a "sudden," major breakthrough. Very motivating!

How to Warm Up

Warming up is just what it sounds like: Your goal is to slightly raise the temperature of your muscles in order to make them more pliable and responsive. By moving around enough to elevate your heart rate slightly and increase the circulation of blood and other fluids to your muscles, you will bring them the heat and nourishment they need to be strong and flexible.

Warming up involves any gentle, rhythmic motion that extends your range or speed of movement beyond its normal parameters, and that you can sustain for about 10 minutes. For example, one simple warm-up would be to go for a brisk walk. Brisk. A stroll won't do it. Remember: "Beyond your normal parameters." A bike ride or swim would also be good. You don't have to go outside if you would rather not. Dancing to your favorite music is a great way to warm up. Shoulder circles, arm raises, gentle leg swings, hip rotations— anything that doesn't feel strenuous, but that causes your breathing to deepen slightly and that perhaps brings on a little perspiration will warm you up adequately.

To be thoroughly prepared, be sure your warm-up includes some movements that use the muscles you plan to stretch or strengthen that day. For example, if you know you will be doing shoulder work, do a few minutes of actions that move the arms and shoulders through a wide, but nonstressful range of motion. It is as though you are "oiling up your joints" in preparation for your workout.

If you can't sing "Happy Birthday" while warming up, you are working too hard. Slow it down. Breathe. Whether walking, swimming, dancing—breathe! Enjoy the sensation of energy as it begins to hum through your body, preparing it to move.

Finding the Lower Body Core

In general, the term "core" refers to the muscles located at the center, or core of your body: the deep abdominal muscles, the perineal, or pelvic floor muscles, and the muscles in the lower back. By actively contracting the abdominal and perineal muscles in toward each other, imagining that they meet at one point, you support the lower back and create a strong, stabilizing base for all movement involving the spine and legs.

When you engage these core muscles, you gain control over the area of your body where the largest, heaviest muscles and bones are located—sometimes referred to as the "center of gravity." By activating core support you create a firm, anchored base against which all the muscles of your lower body can pull as they contract or stretch; this enables you to explore and practice new, challenging exercises by giving you the control that protects you from getting hurt.

Core support also reinforces correct spinal alignment. Your spine, the flexible structure that supports the weight of your entire upper body, attaches to the pelvis. By using the abdominal and perineal muscles to stabilize the pelvis, and building strength in the important muscles of the lower back, your spine will be better able to maintain its weight-supporting "natural" curves.

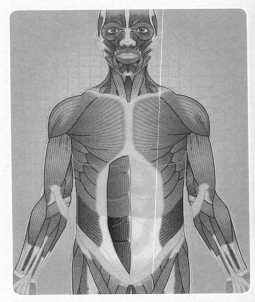

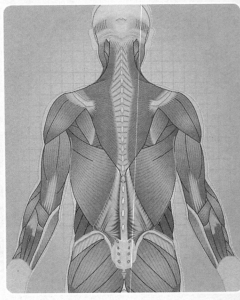

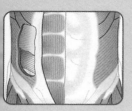

Abdominal Muscles (Transverse Abdominus) This deep, beltlike muscle is the innermost abdominal layer. Unlike the other abdominals, which can bunch up when they contract, the transverse only contracts inward, toward the spine. By engaging it, you will enable all the overlying layers to pull in toward the spine also, creating a strong, flat belly.

Flat Belly Exhale   level: beginning

benefits: Shows how the transverse abdominus can be contracted in order to create core strength.

1   Lie on your back with your knees bent and your feet flat on the floor. Place your hands on the sides of your abdomen, just below the ribs. Inhale slowly, relaxing your belly and allowing it to expand sideways and upward, into your hands.

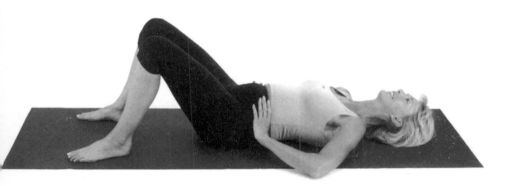

2   Exhale slowly and thoroughly, drawing the abdominals in from all directions in order to squeeze out every last bit of breath. You will feel your waist getting smaller and your belly becoming flat. Repeat 4–6 times.

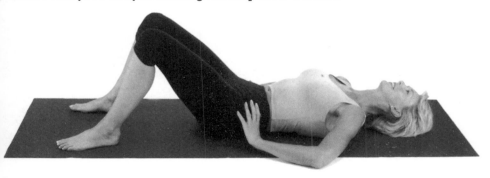

Heel Slide   level: beginning–intermediate

benefits: Trains the core abdominal muscles, or "abs," to stay flat and strong against the counterpull of the legs.

tips: The abdominal muscles are structurally unusual. They are sheathlike and overlay the soft, internal organs, rather than running along rigid bones, as, for instance, the leg and arm muscles do. For this reason, when the superficial layers of abs contract, they can either bunch up and press outward, or pull in, toward the spine. If you allow them to bunch up (as many exercisers make the mistake of doing, when performing the traditional Crunch) you will actually build up a hard and bulbous belly! Hardly your intention, I'm sure. This is why it is so important to learn how to engage the deep core muscles such as the transverse abdominus. ■ These abdominal strengtheners are gentle on the back and safe for most lower back pain sufferers. Of course, check with your doctor before doing any exercise if your back problem is chronic or severe. ■ If you have osteoporosis of the spine, these exercises are safe for you to do. However, abdominal exercises that curl the spine into flexion, such as the Crunch or Bicycle, are not recommended for you.

1 Lie on your back with your knees bent and your feet flat on the floor, arms by your sides. Exhale, pulling the abdominals in toward your spine. (Your lower back needn't touch the floor, but it must remain in a stable position for the entire exercise and not arch up.)

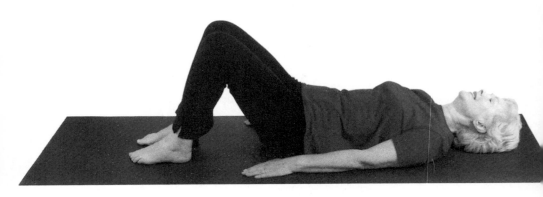

2 Keeping the abdominals strongly engaged, slowly slide the heels forward, as far as you can, keeping the soles of the feet flat and without arching or tensing the back. Stop if you feel the back becoming involved.

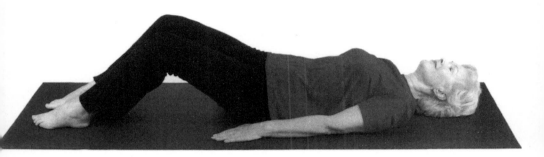

3 Slowly slide your heels back to the start position, keeping your belly muscles "scooped" in and up, and without allowing the back to arch or strain. Rest, take a big "belly breath," then repeat. Repeat 4–8 times.

Variation

If you can't keep from arching your back as you slide the heels forward or back, then try sliding one heel after the other until you build up enough strength to move them both at the same time.

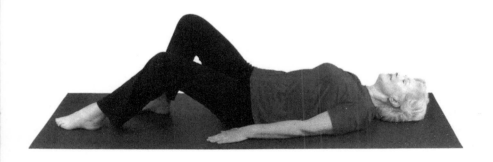

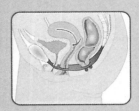

Pelvic Muscles (Perineals) If the pelvis were a box, the abs would be the front of the box, your sacrum the back, and the perineals, the bottom. When contracted, the perineals act with the transverse abdominus to solidify your core support and enhance spinal alignment. Often underdeveloped, these are the muscles that help prevent urinary incontinence.

Kegels level: beginning–advanced

benefits: Strengthens the perineal muscles, which comprise the floor of the pelvis. When you contract these muscles, the abdominal muscles, especially the transverse abdominus, are able to work better.

tips: The perineal muscles of the pelvic floor are flat and shelflike. They are located between the pubic bone and the tailbone. Picture this pelvic floor as an elevator rising from the basement to the roof as you do the Kegels. ■ The perineal muscles are the most underrated muscles in the body. They assist the deep abdominals to contract more strongly, they help with the "Why are the bathrooms so far away all of a sudden?!" problem (what doctors refer to as "urge incontinence"), and they can even encourage your spine to straighten! ■ This last concept is a simple but powerful one. In yoga, the term "mulabanda" is used to describe the pulling in and up of the pelvic floor. By doing so, energy is sent up the spine. Try it right now, as you sit here reading these words. Like a tree growing up from the ground, your spine will lengthen upward into vibrant, strain-free alignment. This is a good tip to keep in mind for those times when you feel down and depleted; it is an instant energy pickup.

1 Imagine that you are urinating and want to stop midstream. Contract the muscles you would use if you were doing this. Try to hold this contraction for a count of "5" then relax. Repeat this 10–20 times, and throughout the day whenever you happen to think of it. You can do this exercise standing or sitting.

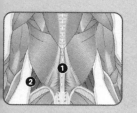

Lower Back Muscles (❶ Erector Spinae and ❷ Quadratus Lumborum) The Erector spinae is a group of several small muscles lying paired on either side of the spine. They extend, or arch the spine, as in a swan dive. Along with the quadratus lumborum and the oblique abdominals, they help stabilize the pelvis, providing core support.

Back Stabilization or Bird Dog

level: beginning

benefits: One of the best beginning level exercises for strengthening the back —especially the lower back—as it learns to maintain its stability.

1 Kneel on the floor, with the hands directly beneath your shoulders and the fingers pointing forward. The knees should be directly beneath the hips and your head, shoulders, and hips should be in a straight line with your nose pointing toward the floor.

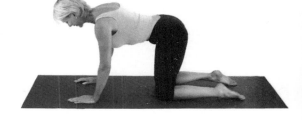

2 Engage your core by firmly contracting the deep abdominal muscles and lifting the pelvic floor; this stabilizes the lower back. Slowly raise the left leg to hip-height. Don't arch the back or allow shoulders to hunch. Hold for about 20 seconds. Breathe! Lower the leg, then repeat on the other side. Repeat 6–8 times, alternating sides.

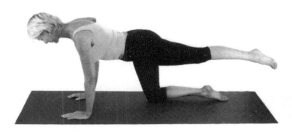

Variation

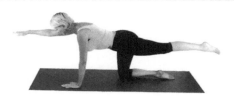

Once you have mastered the exercise, increase the challenge to your core stability by raising the opposite arm forward as you raise the leg. Try to keep the shoulders pulled down away from the ears as you do this. Repeat 6–8 times, alternating sides.

Child's Pose

benefits: Stretches and relaxes the back.

Kneel on the floor with your knees hip-width apart (or wider, if you find that more comfortable), then sit back onto your heels. Relax your upper body forward, resting your forehead on the floor—or on a small pillow, if your head doesn't touch the floor. Place your arms next to your sides. Relax. Breathe deeply and fully. Let go of any tension in your back, shoulders, or anywhere else it may be lodged. Hold this pose for the time it takes to breathe about six deep, slow breaths.

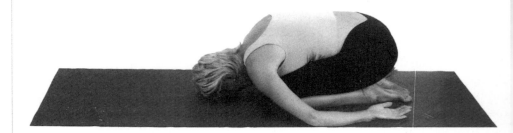

Variation

If it feels better, you may take your arms in front of you and rest them on the floor, palms down. Don't overstretch the arms. Simply relax.

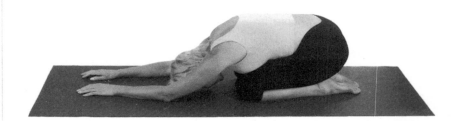

Rock and Roll Stretch

benefits: Another one to stretch and relax the lower back.

tips: This is such a pleasant and relaxing stretch that you may find yourself doing it quite often during your workout. "Rock and Roll" after any exercise that works the muscles on the back of your body, including hamstring, gluteal, lower and upper back strengtheners. By taking the time to rest and stretch, you will help your muscles adjust to the challenge of building strength. ■ This is a wonderful way to relieve stress, whether physical, mental, or emotional. You don't need to be warmed up, because "Rock and Roll" is gentle and safe for the joints and muscles. Simply find a quiet place where you won't be disturbed and use a blanket or mat to cushion your spine. Breathe deeply. Let go of any tension in your neck, shoulders, or wherever else it is lurking. "Rock and Roll" until you feel the stress leave your body.

❶ Lie on your back, bring your knees in toward your chest, and hold behind the knees.

❷ Gently rock an inch or two side to side, relaxing the hip sockets and shoulders as you go. Breathe fully and slowly. Then roll the lower back in small circles, much as you would tilt and roll a small saucer along its edge. Roll 5–6 times in one direction, then reverse directions. This should feel like a nice, relaxing massage for your lower back. Roll over onto your side to get up once you are finished stretching.

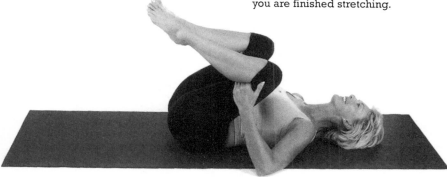

Finding the Upper Body Core

By using the (often weak) muscles of the mid-back to draw the shoulder blades in toward each other and down, away from the ears, you will create a stable muscular base from which to perform all arm movements. You will also achieve beautiful, upright postural alignment. Using some poetic license, we can think of this as the "core support" for the upper body.

This concept is vitally important to over-50s. Slumped upper back posture not only looks awful, it often leads to shoulder or neck pain or rotator cuff (see page 100) injury, and can even contribute to vertebral fractures if you have osteoporosis.

Train yourself to pull your shoulder blades in and down, especially before doing any exercises involving the upper body. You will get the fastest and best results, with least risk of injury.

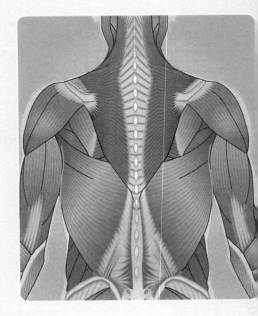

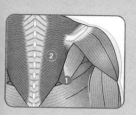

Shoulder and Upper Body Muscles (❶ Rhomboids and ❷ Mid-Trapezius) To correct round shoulders and build a strong upper body core, these are the muscles to work. They contribute to good posture by drawing the scapulae or shoulder blades in toward the spine, creating a stable base for arm and shoulder exercises.

Scapular Squeeze level: beginning

benefits: Strengthens the middle trapezius muscles and the rhomboids, and so helps to create a stabilizing upper body "core."

tips: Be sure to pull the tops of the shoulders down, away from your ears, as you do the scapular squeeze. ▬ This feels great!

1 Stand tall, legs slightly apart with your arms hanging by your sides, palms facing your thighs, then squeeze the shoulder blades, in toward each other. This action will cause your upper arm bones to rotate out, away from the center of your chest. It will also change the orientation of your palms to your body—they might end up facing front. Hold for 5 seconds, then relax. Repeat at least 10 times.

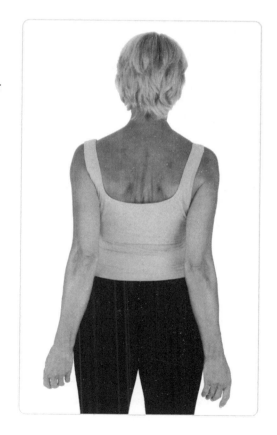

Scapular Squeeze with Weights

level: beginning–intermediate

benefits: Further strengthens the mid-back muscles that comprise the upper body core. Also strengthens the posterior deltoid muscles.

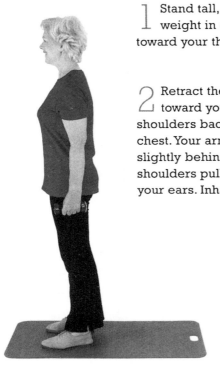

1 Stand tall, with your legs slightly apart and holding a weight in each hand. Make sure that your palms face in toward your thighs.

2 Retract the shoulder blades in toward your spine, drawing the shoulders back and opening the chest. Your arms should now be slightly behind you. Keep your shoulders pulled down, away from your ears. Inhale.

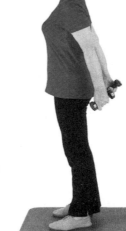

3 Maintaining the position of the shoulder blades, exhale and slowly raise the weights behind you, keeping your arms straight. Stop raising the weights as soon as you feel your shoulders beginning to hunch up or roll forward. Inhale as you lower the weights. Repeat 10–15 times, then repeat the set.

Cat/Cow Stretch

benefits: Stretches the upper and lower back, and allows you to feel how the shoulder blades move on the back ribs.

tips: The more you can coordinate your breathing with the poses, as described below, the better the stretch will be. ■ The upper-arm rotation may feel strange, if not impossible at first. Just keep working at it, as it will be very beneficial for shoulder strengthening and upper-body alignment.

❶ Kneel on the floor, with the hands directly beneath your shoulders and the fingers pointing forward. The knees should be directly beneath the hips and your head, shoulders, and hips should be in a straight line with your nose pointing toward the floor. Slightly rotate your upper arms outward, so that the insides of your elbows face forward.

❷ Inhale as you squeeze the shoulder blades in and reach the sitting bones up and back. At the same time, reach the crown of your head forward and look up slightly. Keep the shoulders pulled down, away from your ears. Hold this position for a moment and enjoy the stretch it gives the front of your body. This is the "cow."

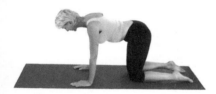

❸ On the exhale, allow the shoulder blades to move apart as you tuck the tailbone under and bring your chin in toward your chest. Use your lower body core strength to draw the abdominal muscles deeply in toward your spine. Your spine will curve up, toward the ceiling, like an angry cat. Feel the stretch distributed throughout the length of the spine. This is the "cat." Return to the "cow" pose, and continue alternating it with the "cat." Do 4–6 sets.

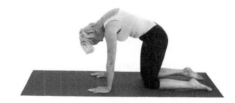

Child's Pose

(page 28)

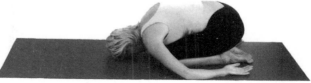

Connecting the Upper and Lower Cores

Now you understand how to activate core support in your lower body, and also how to use the muscles of your mid-back to create a similarly stabilizing base for all upper body movements. These powerful tools will serve you well as you learn how to strengthen your muscles. But what really matters is knowing how to move as a whole person, not a composite of strong and shapely parts!

Here are two simple—but not so easy—exercises to give you an unmistakable sense of connection through your center. You will feel exactly which muscles need to be stretched, and which need to be strengthened, in order to have beautiful, strong, and strain-free spinal alignment. This is an instant "de-slumper."

Use this information to help guide all your strength-building work, and return to these exercises from time to time as a way to measure your progress.

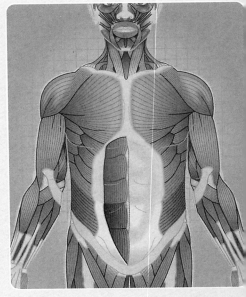

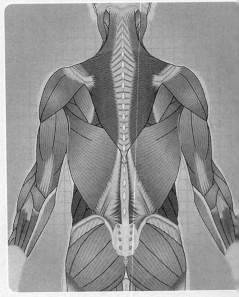

Up against the Wall   level: beginning

benefits: Trains core stability in both the upper and lower body, allowing you to feel clearly how this influences your spinal alignment.

tips: Notice if your belly is sticking out, as it usually does the first time you try this exercise. If this is happening, pull the abdominal and perineal muscles in and up to engage your lower core strength. This will lengthen your lower back into correct, neutral alignment.

1 Stand with your back to a wall, and your heels about 2–3 inches (5–7 cm) away from the wall. Rest your gluteals, the backs of your shoulders, the backs of your hands, and, if possible, the back of your head, against the wall. Retract the shoulder blades in toward each other to open and lift the chest. Hold this position for about 3 breaths. Relax, then repeat the exercise a few more times to strengthen your awareness of how the core muscles interact with each other.

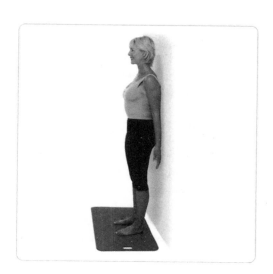

Variation

Stand as described above. Pull the shoulder blades down and in toward the spine as you slowly sweep the arms up and down the wall, as if you were making snow angels. Draw in deep, full breaths as you raise the arms, and exhale as you lower them. Your energy will revive and your shoulders and back will loosen considerably.

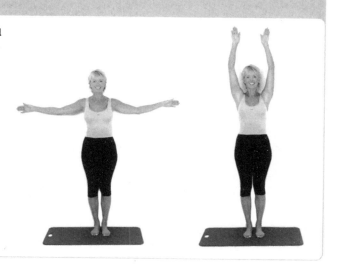

Once you've warmed up, the Squat is a great way to begin your lower body strengthening, whatever your level of fitness. With this one exercise you will begin to build strength in the largest muscles of the lower body—the gluteals, the hamstrings, and the quadriceps. You will be working these muscles in coordination, the way they perform in "real life" (for instance when standing up from a low chair, or descending stairs, or jumping up to reach something). That's what makes the Squat a foundational exercise, along with the fact that it will prepare your muscles for more specifically targeted strengthening work later.

Practice the Squats first. Become familiar with correct form and alignment, especially in your knees and back. Using your core strength will make these weight-bearing exercises both easier and more effective. Variations for more or less challenge are included so you can find the ones that suit you.

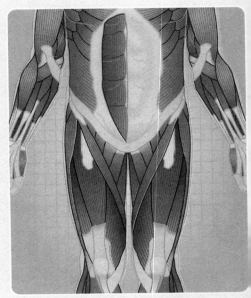

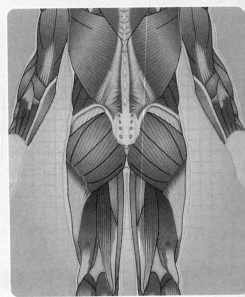

Door Squat   level: beginning

benefits: This will provide all the benefits of the basic Squat, but is a good alternative for those whose balance is "iffy" or who are protecting sensitive knees.

tips: Keep your elbows bent and your shoulders down, away from your ears to avoid straining the shoulders. ▬ Be sure to align your knees directly above the toes.

1 Stand straddling the edge of an open door and grasp a doorknob with each hand. Engage the core muscles and stand tall.

2 Inhale and slowly bend your knees, reaching your gluteals backward, and maintaining an upright position in your chest by squeezing the shoulder blades together. Lower the thighs as close to parallel to the floor as you can, without feeling strain on the knees. Hold for 5 seconds. Exhale as you return to stand. Repeat 6–10 times.

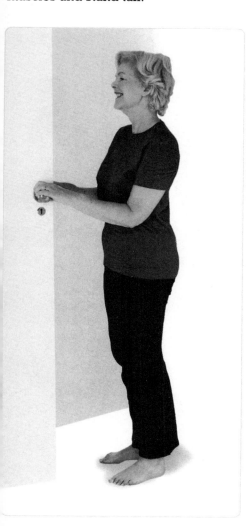

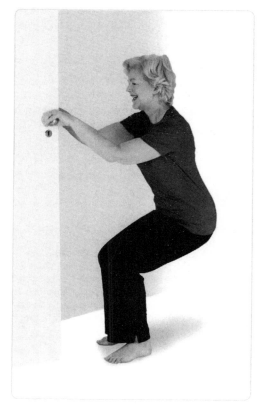

Basic Squat   level: beginning–intermediate

benefits: An excellent exercise, as it builds strength in all the muscles of the lower body, especially the quadriceps muscles and gluteals.

tips: It is important to align the knees correctly. Be sure to keep them pointing directly over your toes, not out to the sides or in toward each other. ■ Don't let the knees move farther forward than the toes as you squat. Keeping your weight backward and into the heels will help you do this correctly. ■ If the Squats still feel too stressful to your knees, then try bending them only one-third of the way.

1 Stand with your feet hip-width apart. Rest a weight on top of each of your shoulders. Activate your lower core muscles.

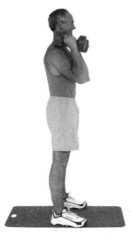

2 Inhale as you slowly bend the knees, shifting your weight backward toward your heels. Keep your chest upright by squeezing the shoulder blades together. Look straight ahead and lower your body until the thighs are nearly parallel to the floor.

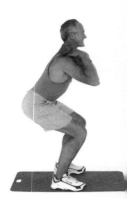

3 Exhale and tighten your gluteals as you straighten your knees, pressing down through the heels to do so. Repeat 10 times, then rest and do another 10.

Variation

Once you can do three sets of 10 basic Squats, you might like to try the much more advanced single-leg Squats. Electromyography shows that this is one of the strongest gluteal strengtheners. Rest a weight on top of each shoulder and activate the core muscles. Follow Steps 2 and 3, above, but hold one foot slightly off the floor as you bend the knees. You don't need to bend the standing knee very much to feel how hard the glutes are working.

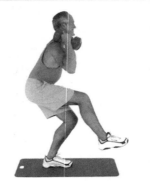

Squats with Stability Ball

level: beginning–intermediate

benefits: Added back support from the ball will make this more comfortable, but also more challenging for the balance.

1 Place a large stability ball against the wall and lean against it with your lower back. Your feet should be hip-width apart and about 2–3 feet (60–90 cm)away from the wall, and your arms should hang by your sides.

2 Inhale as you slowly bend the knees, lowering your body until your thighs are nearly parallel to the floor, if possible. (Your knees shouldn't pass the toes.) Engage the core as you hold this position for about 5 seconds.

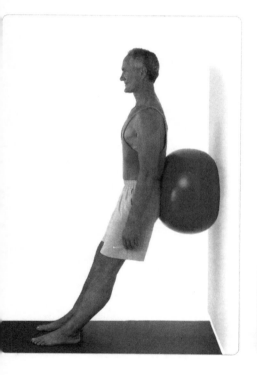
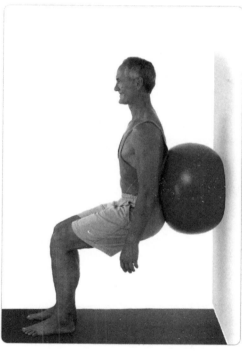

3 Exhale as you tighten the gluteals and press down through the heels in order to straighten the legs. Repeat 10–15 times. Rest, and then repeat the set if desired.

Variation

For extra strengthening, hold weights in your hands as you perform the exercise.

Single Leg Squats with Stability Ball

level: intermediate–advanced

benefits: Strengthens the muscles of the lower body, especially the gluteals and quadriceps. Strengthens balance skills and lower core engagement.

tips: Don't rush! Take your time as you bend and straighten the standing leg.
■ To work your way into this exercise, practice simply shifting the weight over one foot as you hold the Squat, but keep the ball of your other foot resting lightly on the floor for balance.

1 Place a large stability ball against the wall and lean against it with your lower back. Your feet should be hip-width apart and about 2–3 feet (60–90 cm) away from the wall, and your arms should hang by your sides.

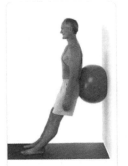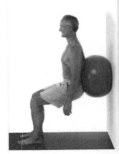

2 Inhale as you slowly bend the knees, lowering your body until your thighs are nearly parallel to the floor, if possible. (Your knees shouldn't pass the toes.) Engage the core as you hold this position for about 5 seconds.

3 Hold your arms out to the sides like a tightrope walker to help you hold your balance, then lift one foot off the ground. Hold the Squat for a breath or two before straightening the standing leg.

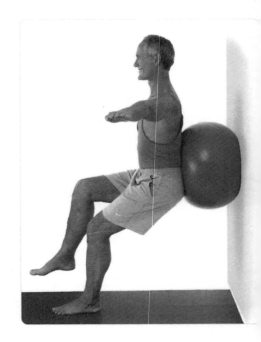

4 Do 6–10 Squats on one leg, then change legs.

Goddess Pose or Wide Plié

level: beginning–advanced

benefits: This strengthens the lower body much as the Squats do, but because the legs are turned out, it provides a slightly different challenge to the muscles —especially the gluteals—as well as to the balance.

tips: Don't allow your bottom to stick out! Focusing on the core muscles will really help. ▬ Try to keep the motion smooth and continuous throughout the exercise. The quality of your movements is as important as the quantity.

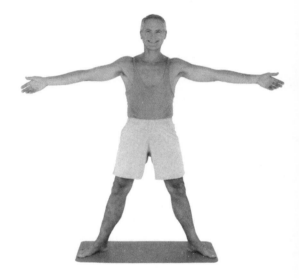

1 Stand with your feet at least shoulder-width apart and turned out about 30–45 degrees. (Your toes will point out to the sides.) Firmly engage your core muscles and raise your arms to just below shoulder height, palms facing forward. Retract your shoulder blades in and relax the shoulders down, away from your ears.

2 Inhale, and slowly bend the knees directly over the toes, until the thighs are as near parallel to the floor as you can manage.

3 Exhale and slowly press down through the heels to straighten your legs. Repeat 6–10 times. Rest and repeat if desired.

Variations

❶ If you find it difficult to raise your arms, work with them by your side.

❷ To make this an advanced exercise, hold the plié position, then lower a little more and hold. Repeat the lower and hold twice more before you straighten the legs.

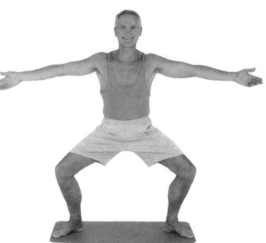

Crossover Stretch

benefits: Stretches the gluteals and the deep hip rotator muscles. Stretches and relaxes the lower back.

tips: Sometimes, especially after you have been sitting too long, the deep rotator muscles of the hip become very tight and cramped. One, in particular, the piriformis, can cause a lot of trouble. That is because it is located so close to the sciatic nerve, the longest nerve in the body. When the piriformis muscle spasms or gets cramped, it can press on the sciatic nerve, causing a dull, toothache-like pain in your lower back and leg. The crossover stretch may help prevent such pain by relaxing the tight piriformis muscle, thus releasing its grip on the sciatic nerve.

❶ Lie on your back with both knees bent and your feet flat on the floor. Rest your arms on the floor next to your body. Place the outside of your right ankle on the top of your bent left knee.

❷ If you are very tight you may get an adequate stretch simply by doing Step 1. You may want to use your hand to press the top knee slightly out to the side, in order to gently increase the stretch.

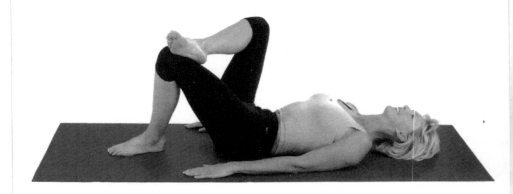

NOTE

This stretch can prevent a flareup of sciatic pain, but only if a tight piriformis muscle is the source of the discomfort. Muscle tension is just one of several possible causes of sciatic pain. If you are experiencing such pain chronically, don't stretch until you see your doctor and learn if it is safe for you to stretch.

❸ Raise your left foot and use your left leg to push both legs in toward your chest. Circle the left, underneath knee 5 times in one direction, and then 5 times in the opposite direction.

❹ Return the left foot to the floor, uncross the legs, and repeat on the other side.

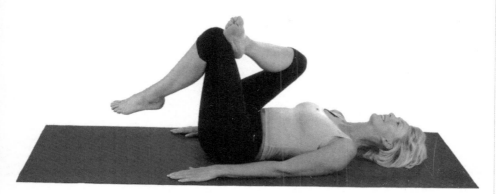

Variation

For a stronger stretch, reach through the legs and grasp the back of your left thigh with both hands. Gently pull the left leg toward you to create a stretch in your right hip and gluteals. Hold for at least 20 seconds. Check to be sure your lower back, shoulders, and neck are also soft and relaxed. You may want to rock slightly side to side; this helps the muscles let go. Repeat on the other side.

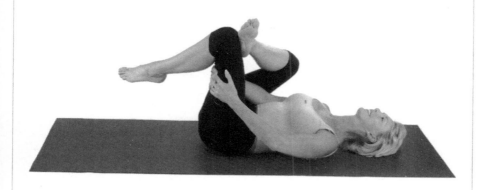

foundational exercises for lower body strength   **43**

Foundational Exercises for Upper Body Strength—The Push-Up

Like the Squats, Push-Ups train the muscles to work in coordination, the way they do when performing the actions of daily life, such as pushing furniture around, or pushing a stroller, or carrying a heavy bag of groceries. They are an efficient and effective exercise for the upper body, but are so often performed wrong that they merit a close look. Activating your upper core support by retracting the shoulder blades toward each other will have a major impact on making the Push-Ups a quick and powerfully strengthening exercise. So will using the stabilizing power of your lower body's core. The following three Push-Ups progressively build foundational strength in your upper body.

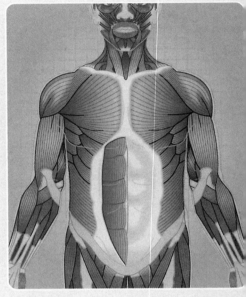

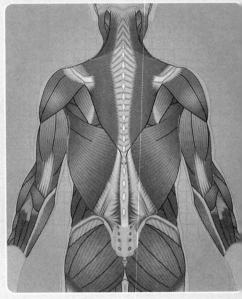

Wall Push-Ups   level: beginning

benefits: A smart way to begin building strength in the chest, shoulder, and arms. This exercise doesn't require weights or getting down on the floor, so you can fit it into even the most streamlined schedule.

1 Stand at about arm's length away from a wall, with your feet hip-width apart. Place your hands on the wall slightly below shoulder height and about shoulder distance apart. (Your heels may or may not leave the floor; either way is fine.) Pull your shoulders down and engage your upper core by retracting the shoulder blades. Activate your lower core by pulling the abdominals in and lifting the floor of the pelvis. Maintain this form for the entire exercise.

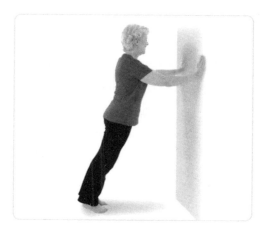

2 Inhale as you slowly bend the elbows.

3 Exhale as you slowly straighten the elbows. Repeat 10 times, then rest. Work up to doing three sets of 10, then you can move on to Knee Push-Ups (page 46).

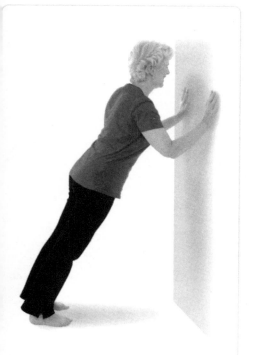

Variation

Once in awhile, place your hands farther apart to work the outer chest more. With the hands closer together, you will work the triceps (back of the arms) more. This kind of alteration of position keeps your muscles "surprised;" they will get stronger faster and will burn more energy than if you always do the same thing. This suggestion applies to the Knee Push-Ups (page 46) and the Full Push-Ups (page 47), as well.

Knee Push-Ups   level: beginning–intermediate

benefits: Increased challenge, but safe and totally doable if you use core strength to stabilize the upper and lower body.

tips: Place a folded towel under your knees if they feel uncomfortable. ■ The lower core is working hard here, but also be sure to maintain a strong position in the upper back by squeezing the shoulder blades in and pulling them down away from your ears.

1 Kneel on all fours. Walk your hands forward until you make a straight line from your ears to your shoulders to your knees. Pull your abdominals in and up to support your back.

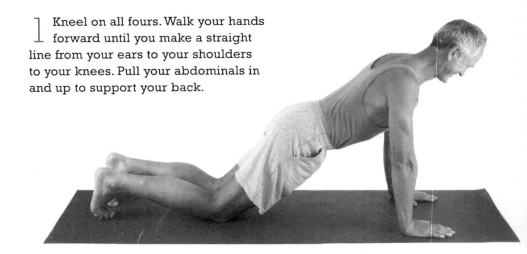

2 Inhale, slowly bending your elbows and lowering your chest toward the floor. Lower only as far as you can while maintaining correct alignment in the back.

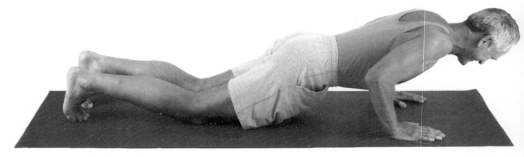

3 Exhale, slowly straightening the arms. Repeat 10 times. Rest, and repeat. When you can complete three sets without losing form, you can move on to Full Push-Ups (opposite).

Full Push-Ups   level: intermediate–advanced

benefits: This is a nearly perfect upper body exercise. If you have been diligent in preparing your muscles for the full push-ups, you will find them challenging but not too unpleasant. These build strength in a hurry!

tips: Do not lock the elbows when doing push-ups to avoid injury. ■■ Firming your leg muscles will help you maintain a solid sense of form and distribute the work throughout your body. ■■ The lowering phase of the push-up is when most of the strength building occurs. Don't rush it!

1 Kneel on all fours. Reach one leg back at a time, tucking the toes under. Straighten your arms and place the hands below the shoulders, fingers pointing straight ahead. Ears, shoulders, hips, and knees should be in one line.

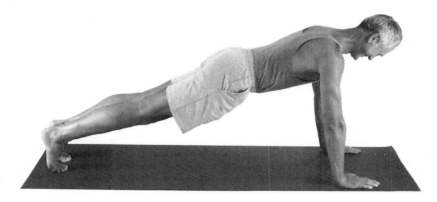

2 Ensuring that your core is active throughout, inhale, bending your elbows out to the sides to a 90-degree angle as you lower your chest toward the floor.

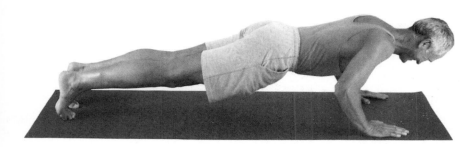

3 Exhale, pushing down into the floor to straighten the arms. Repeat 10 times, then rest and repeat the set. Work up to doing three sets, then reward yourself for a job well done.

Step through the Door Stretch

benefits: This is a simple way to get a great stretch in your chest and front shoulder muscles. No equipment is necessary, other than an open doorway.

tips: Be sure to relax the shoulders down away from the ears. Because it lengthens out the often chronically tight front shoulder muscles, this stretch will help your body perform shoulder blade retraction more easily, too. ▪▪ If you keep the back leg straight and the back heel flat on the floor, you will get a good calf muscle stretch as a bonus.

❶ Stand with right leg forward and left leg back in front of an open door, close enough to rest your forearms on the side frame. Place your elbows at shoulder height, or a little lower, and place the palms, fingers pointing up, flat against the frame.

❷ Step through the door, bending the right knee, until you feel a good stretch in the shoulders and chest. Hold for at least 20 seconds, breathing and relaxing. Repeat on the other side.

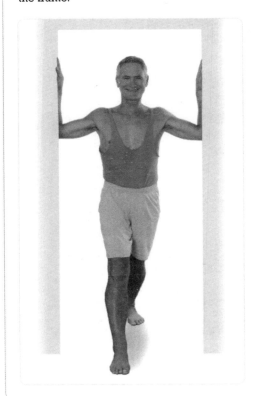
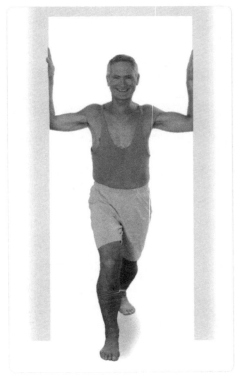

Supine Chest Stretch

tips: Follow this stretch by lying flat on the floor for a moment and breathing easily and softly. Chief benefit? You'll feel fantastic, both relaxed and energized. Bend the knees and roll onto your side to stand when you are done.

① Sit on the stability ball, then walk your feet forward until you are comfortably balanced on top of the ball with your head and entire spine supported (see page 114). Open the arms out to the sides, like a letter "T," with the palms facing upward. Relax and take at least 8 deep breaths. When you are done, hold the ball with both hands and slowly roll yourself forward to end seated on the floor.

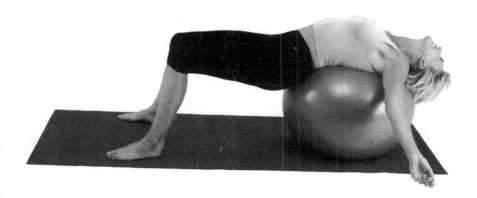

Variation

① After relaxing for a few minutes with your arms out to the sides, slowly move your arms back, until you feel a different (probably stronger) stretch in the chest and shoulder muscles. Continue to breathe deeply, allowing the arms to hang loosely from the shoulders. You may only need to move the arms a very small distance to create this new stretch.

② If you don't have access to a stability ball, you can improvise a similar, supported stretch in the following way. Place a large, firm pillow under your upper back, in such a way that when you recline over it and open your arms to the sides, you feel a stretch in your shoulders and chest. If necessary, use a second pillow under your head so that your neck is comfortably supported and not overly arched. Bend your knees, placing the feet flat on the floor. Breathe and relax for several minutes, then roll to the side to slowly stand up.

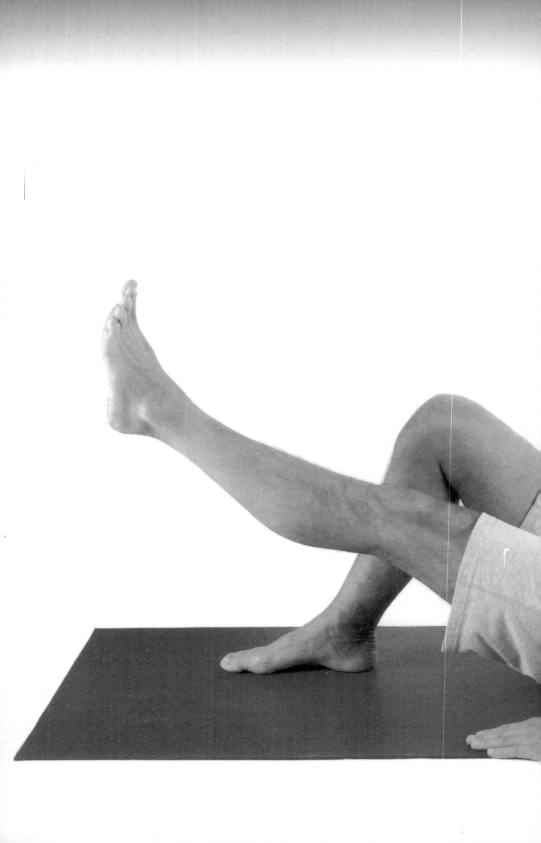

Crossover Stretch
(page 42)

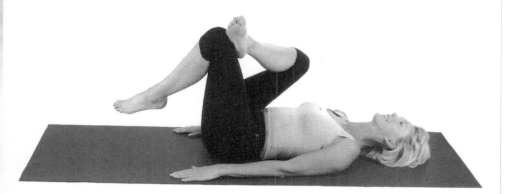

Child's Pose
(page 28)

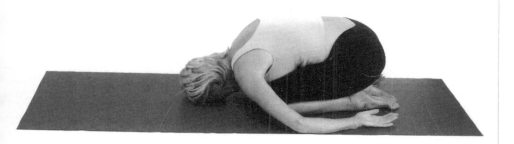

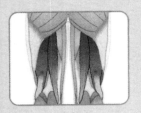

Back of Thigh Muscles (Hamstrings) These thick, strong muscles provide strength and power for walking and running, and help stabilize the pelvis. Be sure to stretch them often: If they are very tight (and, for men especially, they usually are) they can contribute to lower back stiffness and pain.

Hamstring Curls

level: beginning–intermediate

benefits: This is a classic exercise for strengthening the hamstring muscles in the back of the thigh.

1 Kneel on all fours then rest your weight on your forearms with the arms parallel to each other. Draw your shoulders down away from your ears, and pull in the abdomen and pelvic floor, engaging the core. Reach the right leg back to hip height, with the knee facing down toward the floor.

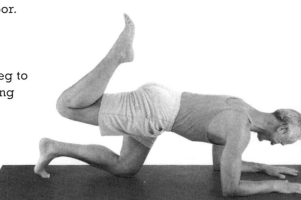

2 Without allowing the right leg to drop, bend the knee, bringing the heel in toward your bottom.

Variation

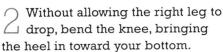

You may clasp the hands together if that is more comfortable.

3 Press the right heel back to straighten the leg. Repeat 10–20 times, then repeat on the other side. Rest, and do one or two more sets.

Arabesque with Curls

level: intermediate–advanced

benefits: This exercise incorporates lower body alignment in a dynamic way. It also offers an opportunity to practice core support under more challenging conditions.

tips: Firmly contract your abs in and up. This will support your lower back and help to solidify your balance.

1 Stand holding the back of a chair for support, arms slightly bent. Engage the lower core and lift the right leg a few inches off the floor behind you; your body should tilt forward from the hips a little, but keep the chest lifted and open. The right knee should face down toward the floor and both hips should be square to the front.

2 Maintain this position as you curl the right heel in toward your bottom.

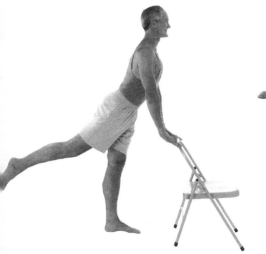 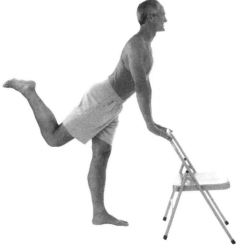

Variation

Once you've mastered this, try doing it without holding onto a support.

3 Stretch the heel back out to straighten the leg. Repeat 10–20 times, then change sides.

Standing Hamstrings Stretch

benefits: Lengthens the hamstrings without straining the lower back.

tips: Don't allow your upper back to round. ■ A little goes a long way in this stretch. Focus on where you feel the stretch; it doesn't matter how far forward your body is tilted.

❶ Stand facing a low chair, or steps, or other sturdy support, and place your hands on your hips. Prop your left heel on the support, keeping your hips squared to the front, and straighten the left knee without locking it. Lift your lower core muscles and look straight ahead.

❷ Keeping your chest lifted and open, tilt forward from the hips until you feel a stretch in the back of the thigh. You won't need to go far! Keep a slight forward curve in your lower back to protect it from strain. Stay here and breathe deeply and slowly for 6–8 breaths. Repeat on the other side.

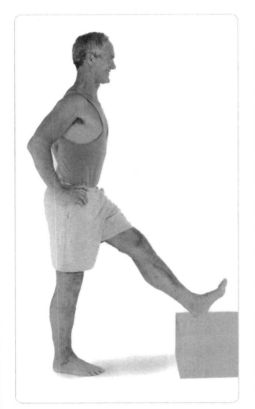

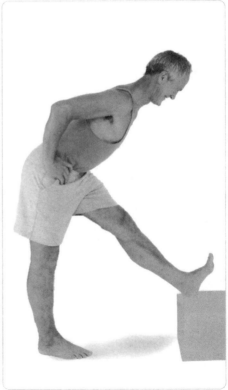

Supine Hamstrings Stretch

benefits: Relaxes and stretches the back as the hamstrings stretch out.

tips: This is an important stretch to do on a regular basis if lower back stiffness is a problem for you.

❶ Lie on your back with knees bent and feet flat on the floor. Lift the right leg and hold onto the back of it just below the knee. Keeping it slightly bent, use your hands to slowly pull the thigh in toward your body until you feel a stretch. Draw your shoulders down, away from your ears. Hold and breathe for about 10 breaths. Rest and repeat on the other side.

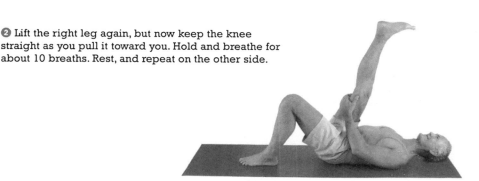

❷ Lift the right leg again, but now keep the knee straight as you pull it toward you. Hold and breathe for about 10 breaths. Rest, and repeat on the other side.

Variation

If you cannot hold the back of your leg without hunching the shoulders, then loop a soft belt or tie over the foot and use that to draw the leg closer.

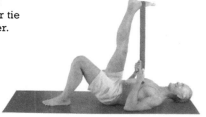

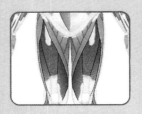

Front of Thigh Muscles (Quadriceps) The quads are the muscles that provide climbing and descending power, as when climbing up or down stairs or getting in and out of chairs. The following are "must do" exercises to strengthen the support of your knee joints.

Tighten and Hold   level: beginning

benefits: Safely strengthens the quadriceps muscles without straining the knee joint.

1 Lie on your back with your arms slightly away from your sides. Place a small stability ball, rolled towel, or small firm pillow beneath the left knee and bend the right leg, placing the foot flat on the floor.

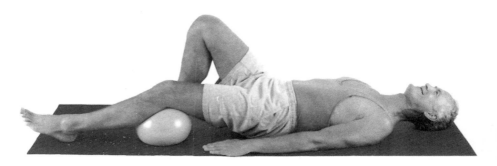

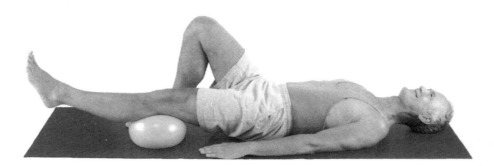

2 Press the left knee into the prop beneath it, feeling the quad muscles firming. Your heel will leave the floor. Hold for five seconds.

3 Relax the quads and lower the heel to the floor. Perform 15–20 times. Rest, then repeat on other side. Repeat the set.

Supine Leg Lift   level: beginning–intermediate

benefits: Strengthens quads and abdominal core muscles at the same time. This can be progressed by gradually adding weight.

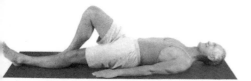

1 Lie on your back with your arms slightly away from your sides. Bend the right leg, placing the foot flat on the floor. Lengthen the left leg forward.

2 Firmly engage your lower core, stabilizing the lower back so it doesn't arch or strain. Lift the left leg about 10 inches (25 cm) off the floor. Hold for 5 seconds, then slowly return the leg to the floor. Repeat 10–20 times, then rest and repeat on the other side. Repeat the set once or twice more.

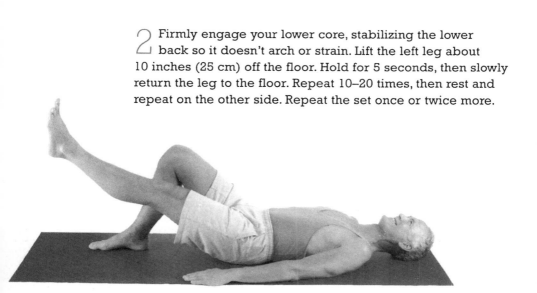

Variations

❶ To make this even more strengthening, don't completely return the leg to the floor, but stop at just an inch above before raising the leg back up.

❷ For the second set, try turning out the working leg at the hip, so that the inner thigh faces the ceiling. This will target the medial quadricep, further strengthening the knee joint.

❸ Try holding a small weight against the thigh of the straight leg.

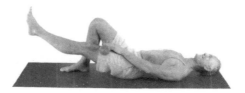

Squats with Stability Ball

level: beginning–intermediate

benefits: The quads get a good workout from this exercise as well.

1 Follow the instructions on page 39 to perform this exercise as part of your quads workout.

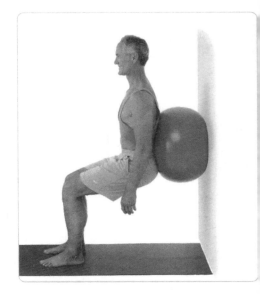

Follow the instructions on page 39

FOLLOW-UP STRETCH

Quads Stretch

tips: If you find it too difficult to grasp the ankle behind you, try looping a soft belt or tie around the ankle. ▬ This shouldn't cause any knee discomfort. If it feels wrong, check to be sure that the knee is in line with the hip and not pointing up or down.

❶ Lie on your left side with both knees bent. Rest your head on the left arm. Stack the shoulders one above the other, and do the same with the hips. Use the core muscles to hold this form.

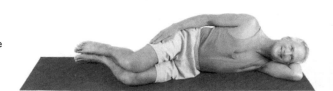

❷ Reach back with your right hand and grasp the right ankle. Gently pull the right foot toward your bottom to create a stretch in the front of the right thigh. Hold the stretch for about 6–10 breaths. Roll onto your back and rest, and then repeat the stretch on the other side.

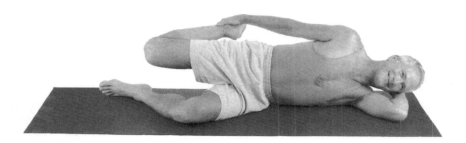

Variation

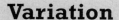

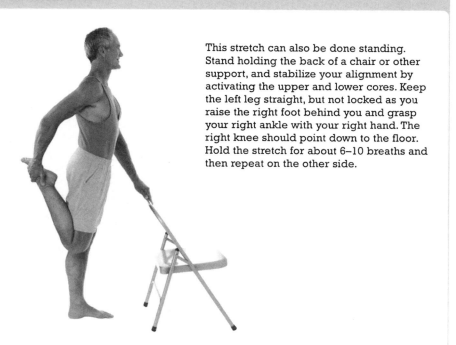

This stretch can also be done standing. Stand holding the back of a chair or other support, and stabilize your alignment by activating the upper and lower cores. Keep the left leg straight, but not locked as you raise the right foot behind you and grasp your right ankle with your right hand. The right knee should point down to the floor. Hold the stretch for about 6–10 breaths and then repeat on the other side.

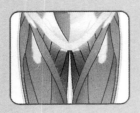

Inner Thigh Muscles (Adductors) These muscles help to navigate twists and turns by providing stability for the legs and pelvis when you move sideways or diagonally. They contribute to balance, and strengthening them will help you fit into those tight pants, too.

Side-Lying Leg Lift for Adductors

level: beginning–advanced

benefits: This strengthens the inner thigh muscles, and helps train lower core strength, too. Simple, safe, and as challenging as you care to make it; just increase the number of repetitions or add some weight.

tips: You must keep your core muscles active at all times to prevent the back from rounding into faulty alignment as you lift the leg.

1 Lie on your left side. Bend your right knee and place the right foot flat on the floor in back of the left leg. Rest your head on the left arm. Lengthen your body, creating a straight line from your ear, to your shoulder, to your hip, to the left leg.

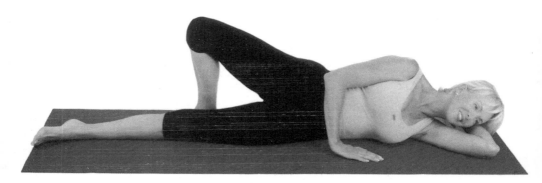

2 Lift the left leg as high as you can, keeping the left knee facing straight ahead, like a headlight on a car. Hold the lift for five seconds, and then lower the leg. Repeat 10–20 times. Rest. Repeat on other side. Repeat the set.

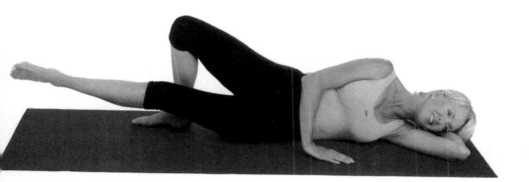

Variations

❶ The exercise can be performed with the foot of the bent leg resting on the floor in front of the straight leg, if that feels more balanced and comfortable to you.

❷ Try this exercise with an ankle weight on the lower leg. Be sure to keep the knee straight to prevent strain or injury to it when using weights.

❸ Even without using an ankle weight, you can instantly increase the level of difficulty in the following way: once you have lifted the leg as high as you can, lift it just an inch more, then lower it an inch. Repeat this small but intense "pulsing" action 5–10 times. Lower the leg to the floor, and repeat 10 more times.

❹ Here is another way of increasing the level of difficulty. While the leg is lifted, "draw" small circles in the air with the heel. Keep the knee straight and move the leg away from the hip. Do 5–10 circles in one direction, then reverse directions. Lower the leg, then repeat 10 more times.

The Scissors   level: beginning–advanced

benefits: An efficient exercise, as it strengthens the adductors of both legs at once, while also providing an opportunity to strengthen the lower abdominal muscles.

tips: This will stretch the adductors as well as strengthen them, and that may be what you notice most! ■ Prevent injury or strain to the hips and adductors by being sure to avoid using momentum as you open the legs to the sides.

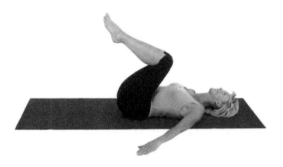

1 Lie on your back, with your knees drawn in toward your chest and your arms resting on the floor slightly away from the sides of the body, palms facing down.

2 Reach your feet toward the ceiling, keeping the legs parallel to each other, and slightly bent if necessary. Activate your lower core by pulling the deep abdominal muscles in and the pelvic floor up.

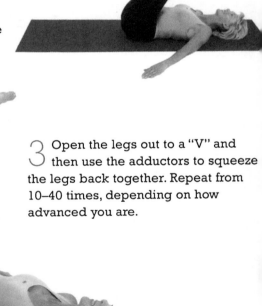

3 Open the legs out to a "V" and then use the adductors to squeeze the legs back together. Repeat from 10–40 times, depending on how advanced you are.

Wall Sit with Ball between the Knees

level: beginning–advanced

benefits: Pressing a small ball between the knees makes this Squat variation especially strengthening for the adductors.

tips: A firm pillow squeezed between the knees will work just as well as a ball.

1 Stand with your back against a wall and your feet hip-width apart. Walk your feet 2–3 feet (60–90 cm) away from the wall and place a small ball (10–12 inches/25–30 cm) between your legs, just above the knees.

2 Inhale as you slowly bend the knees, bringing them as close to a 90-degree angle as is comfortable. (The knees shouldn't pass the toes.) Engage the lower body core and squeeze the ball between your knees, holding the squeeze for about 5 seconds.

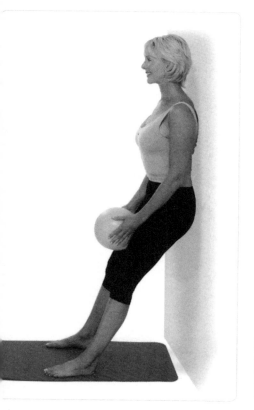
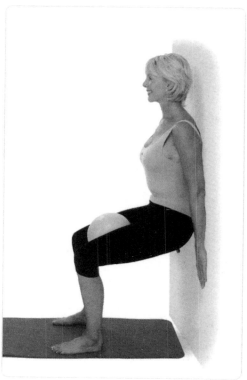

3 Exhale as you tighten the gluteals and press down through the heels in order to straighten the legs. Repeat 10 times, then rest. Repeat the set if desired.

The Potted Plant

tips: If you cannot sit straight, then place a firm cushion beneath your buttocks; this will elevate the pelvis and free up the hips.

❶ Sit with the soles of the feet together and hands on the floor slightly behind you to help you sit straight. Lengthen your back into good alignment, with the ears above the shoulders, above the hips. Allow your shoulders to relax down, away from your ears. Breathe for about 4–6 deep breaths.

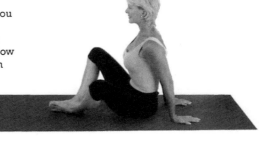

❷ To deepen the stretch, hold above the ankles and lean forward slightly from the hips. Rest the elbows on the knees and keep the chest open so that the upper back doesn't round. Hold and breathe for about 6–8 deep breaths.

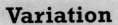

Variation

If this stretch feels strenuous, try doing it with your back flat against a wall, for support. It will be just as effective, perhaps even more so, because you will be comfortable enough to relax more deeply.

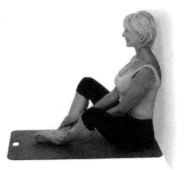

Standing Adductor Stretch with Plié

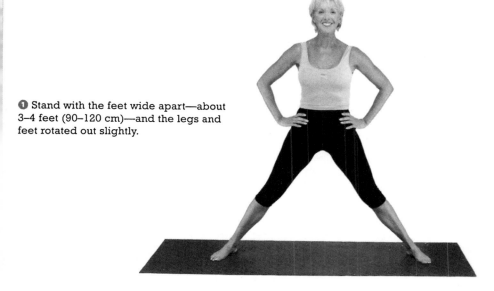

❶ Stand with the feet wide apart—about 3–4 feet (90–120 cm)—and the legs and feet rotated out slightly.

❷ Hinge forward from your hips, bending the right knee directly over the right foot, and resting your hands on the top of your thighs for balance. Keep your body centered between the legs, rather than letting it move toward the bent knee. You will feel a stretch, especially in the left leg. Hold for about three or four deep breaths, then slowly straighten the right leg.

❸ Repeat, bending the other knee. Repeat as often as you feel is necessary to get the benefits of the stretch.

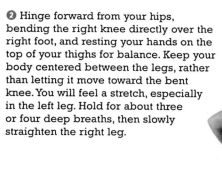

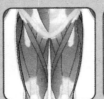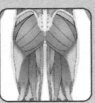

Outer Thigh Muscles (Abductors) These are the muscles that pull the thighs away from each other. They are extremely important for their contribution to balance, stabilizing the pelvis, and esthetics.

Side-Lying Leg Lift for Abductors

level: beginning–advanced

benefits: Simple, but not easy strengthener for the outer thigh muscles. This exercise will allow you to build strength gradually and to work intensively without risking injury.

tips: This exercise feels like nothing much at first. Don't worry; it adds up quickly once the abductor begins to "get the message."

1 Lie on your left side, with your shoulders and hips vertically stacked, and your head resting on your left arm. Rest your right hand on the floor in front of your chest and bend the left (underneath) leg so the knee is facing forward, for balance. Straighten the right leg, firming the quadriceps muscles above the knee. Your body should form a straight line, from the ears through the shoulders, hips, right knee, and right ankle.

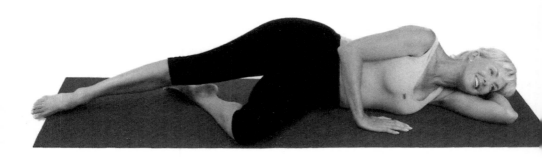

2 Lift the right leg about 12 inches (30 cm), keeping the knee directed straight forward.

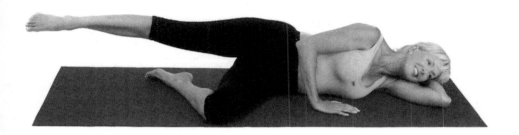

3 Lower the right leg to just above the left leg. Repeat 10–20 times, rest, then change sides. Repeat the set once or twice more.

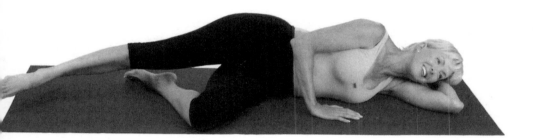

Variation

You may add a weight for further challenge. Hold it against the top thigh to avoid possible strain to your knee.

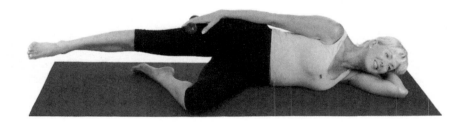

Pizza Circles   level: beginning–intermediate

benefits: Moves the upper leg through a full 360 degrees, strengthening the abductor muscles from all angles.

1 Lie on your left side with both knees bent, resting one upon the other. Vertically stack the shoulders and hips. Activate your core to maintain this position throughout the exercise. Your back should be in neutral alignment, with the head and shoulders in line with the hips. Place your right hand on the floor in front of your waist for stability.

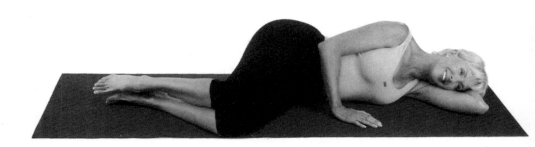

2 Lift the right leg until the thigh is parallel to the floor, and bring the right knee forward toward your nose.

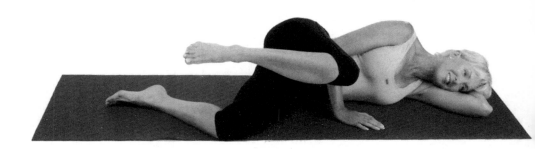

3 Circle the right knee up toward the ceiling, keeping the knee facing forward as much as you can.

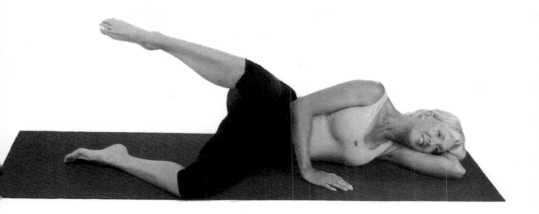

4 Circle the right knee back away from your head, continuing around in the same direction. It is as if you were using the knee to trace the perimeter of a large pizza balancing on its edge. Do 5–10 circles in one direction, then reverse the direction. Rest. Roll onto your back, and then do the other side. Repeat the set . . . if you can!

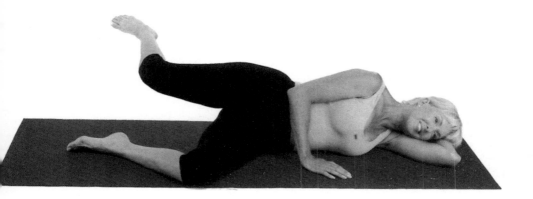

Front and Back Swing

level: intermediate–advanced

benefits: This requires close attention to core stabilization, as it helps you feel how the abductors work through a large range of movement.

tips: It is often difficult to keep the swinging leg at the same height throughout, but doing so will truly work those abductors. ■■ In order to keep the top leg level as it moves forward and back of your body, imagine you are sliding it over a very low table.

1 Lie on your left side with the left arm extended, your right hand on the floor in front of your waist for stability and the right leg resting on the left leg. Make sure that shoulders and hips are vertically stacked, your back is in neutral alignment, and the knees are facing straight ahead.

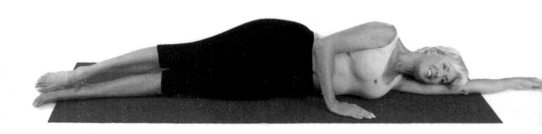

2 Lift the right leg just to hip height.

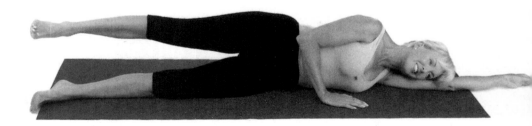

3 Strongly engage the core muscles in the upper and lower body to keep the body still as you slowly swing the right leg forward and back, keeping it level. This is one swing. Be sure to keep the left knee facing front. Use the core to prevent the lower back from arching or the shoulders from tilting. Do 6–10 swings, then change sides.

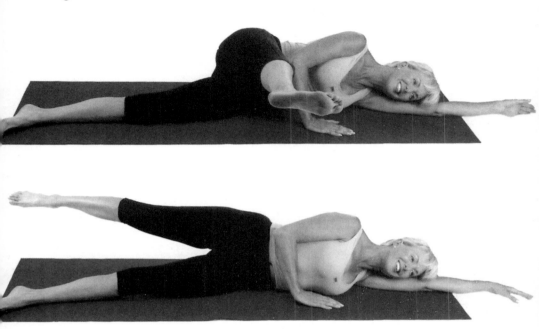

FOLLOW-UP STRETCH

Crossover Stretch

(page 42)

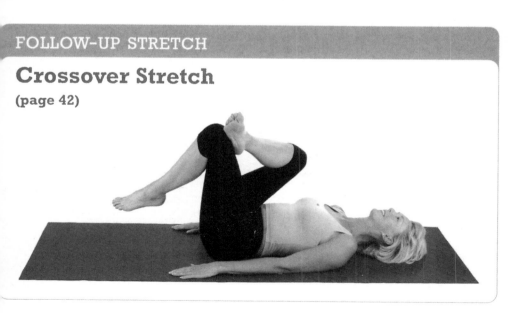

Spiral Stretch

benefits: Stretches the outer thigh and hip muscles. Also stretches the spine and chest.

❶ Lie on your back with both knees bent and pressed gently together, and the feet flat on the floor. Rest your arms on the floor straight out to the sides, like a letter "T."

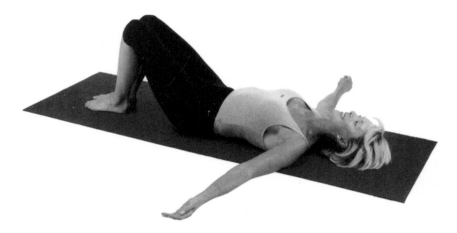

❷ Slowly lower the knees to the right; turning your head to the left at the same time. Relax into the stretch for at least 6–10 deep, slow breaths, then bring the knees back to the center and slowly lower them to the other side, changing the position of your head, too. Repeat this stretch as many times as you'd like.

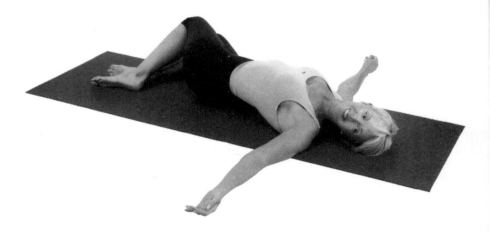

Variations

❶ Try pressing down on the top knee with the opposite hand to create a stronger stretch.

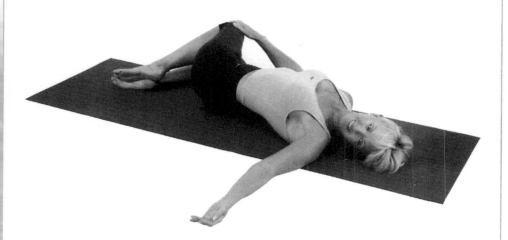

❷ Try bringing the knees into your chest before lowering them to the floor. This will change the location of the stretch and may feel stronger.

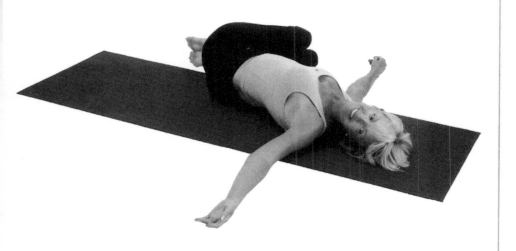

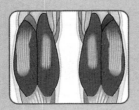

Calf Muscles (Gastrocnemius) These are the muscles that provide "push-off power" when we are walking, running, and jumping. They have substantial impact on strengthening your balance, too. Stretch them every day if you wear heels or are a runner.

Heel Raises   level: beginning-advanced

benefits: A simple yet effective "gastroc" strengthener.

1 Stand facing the back of a chair or other sturdy support, resting the hands on it for balance and having your legs hip-width apart. The shoulders should be relaxed and the lower core engaged. Raise the heels, pressing them directly forward toward the second toe to ensure proper ankle alignment. Hold for 5 seconds, then lower. Repeat 10–20 times. Rest, and repeat.

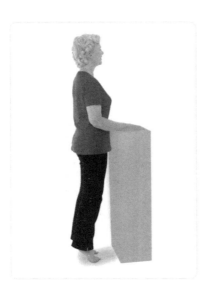

Variations

❶ To advance the pose, try resting one foot behind the ankle of the other one, and do the raises on one foot at a time.

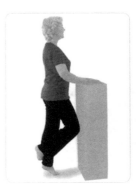

❷ Stand with the front of both feet on a step, and your heels hanging down.

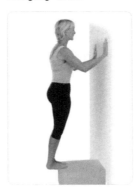

❸ From this stretched position, raise the heels to their full height.

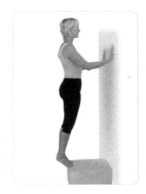

Gastrocnemius Stretch or Runners' Stretch

❶ Stand at about arm's length away from a wall. Place your hands on the wall slightly above shoulder height and about shoulder distance apart. Bend the left knee directly over the foot, keeping most of your weight into that foot, as you take a large step back with your right foot. Keep your body in a straight line with the right leg, from ear to ankle. Keep the chest lifted, even though the upper body will be slightly tilted forward. Check to see that both legs are parallel, not turned out. The back heel should not be touching the floor.

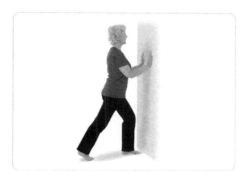

❷ Keeping the right leg very straight, slowly press the right heel toward the floor, until you feel a stretch in the calf muscle. Hold this stretch for about 4–6 breaths.

❸ Straighten the left leg and, keeping the right heel pressed down into the floor, bend the right knee. This will move the stretch to the soleus muscle, just above the heel. Hold the stretch for about 4–6 breaths, then repeat both stretches on the other side.

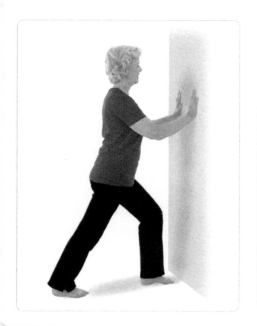

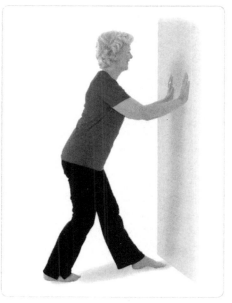

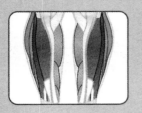

Shin Muscles (Dorsi Flexors) These muscles pull the toes up, away from the floor, which is especially important for the much-older-than-50s, as it prevents the foot drop (shuffling) that often occurs in the unexercised older population. This is a major cause of falls.

Ankle Flex against Resistance

level: beginning

benefits: Strengthens the muscles that lift the front of the foot, enabling one to step heel first.

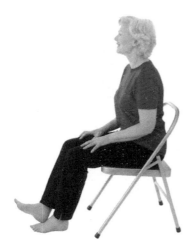

1 Sit comfortably on a chair and place the left foot flat on the floor, its ankle directly beneath the knee if possible. Place the heel of the right foot on the instep of the left foot. Relax the right leg, so that its weight rests on the left foot.

2 Flex the left foot at the ankle so its heel remains on the floor but its toes point up toward the ceiling, at the same time resisting that action with the weight of the right foot. Hold this position for 5 seconds, then relax the flex. Repeat 10–15 times, then change feet.

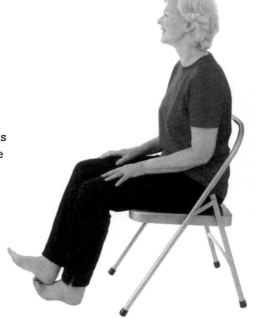

Foot Point Stretch

tips: By manually manipulating the foot, you will create a good stretch and avoid the painful foot and toe cramps that sometimes accompany this toe-pointing movement. If by chance you do get a cramp, don't panic: simply stretch your toes in the opposite direction and the cramp will go away. ▬ This stretch will help relieve painful "shin splints." ▬ While you are at it, why not use your hands to circle the foot around at the ankle and to massage the tight, sore spots on the bottom, sides, or top of the foot? This doesn't just feel great: it also increases flexibility and circulation.

Sit comfortably on a chair and cross the right leg over the left, so that the right foot is hanging loosely. Holding the right ankle, use the other hand to firmly grasp the front of the right foot and stretch it into a pointed position, like a ballet dancer. Still using your hands, curl the toes under, toward the sole of your foot, pressing only as much as feels good. Relax, then repeat. Do this for a few minutes, then change sides.

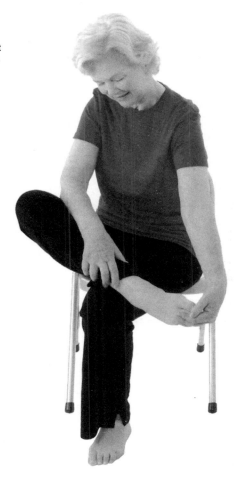

Strengthening the Upper Body

The following exercises will continue the strengthening work that Push-Ups began, by targeting the shoulder and arm muscles in a more focused way. Begin by working the large muscles in the front of the upper body, the chest and shoulders, and follow that with some strengtheners for your upper back and rear shoulders. (These exercises are particularly good for your posture.) The next front/back pairing of muscles, the triceps and biceps are fun to work on because they can bring such fast, visible results: very motivating!

The last section will teach you how to strengthen the rotator cuff muscles, the muscles that attach the upper arm to the back. Problems with these muscles are endemic to the over-50s, especially the weekend warrior types, who suddenly decide to rake the lawn or play singles tennis after not having done so in a long time. These simple rotator cuff exercises may prevent such notoriously slow-healing injuries from occurring.

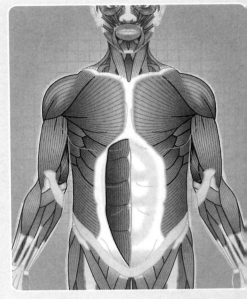

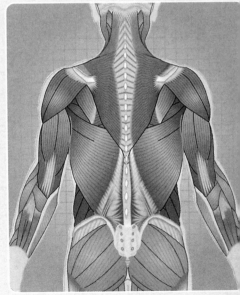

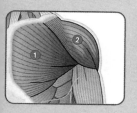

Chest Muscles (❶ Pectorals) and Front of Shoulder Muscles (❷ Anterior Deltoids) These are the muscles that provide pushing power—and that give a nice shape to the chest.

Chest Fly with Weights

level: beginning–advanced

benefits: Strengthens the chest and front shoulders.

tips: In this and any exercise involving weights, be sure to lift and lower the weights slowly: avoid using momentum. It should take at least 6 seconds to complete one repetition.

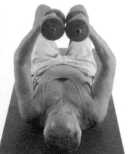

1 Lie on the floor with both knees bent and the feet flat. Holding a weight in each hand, palms facing each other, press the weights up above the center of your chest, drawing your shoulders down away from your ears and in toward each other. Slightly round your elbows, and keep them rounded this way throughout the exercise.

2 Inhale, and slowly open the arms out to the sides, stopping before they reach shoulder level. Exhale and slowly pull the arms back up to the starting position. Repeat 10–15 times. Rest and repeat the set once or twice more.

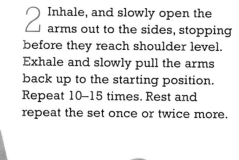

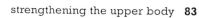

Spiral Stretch (page 76)

tips: Be sure to keep your shoulders flat on the floor in order to get the best chest stretch.

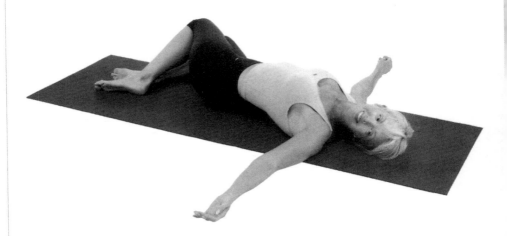

Supine Chest Stretch
(page 49)

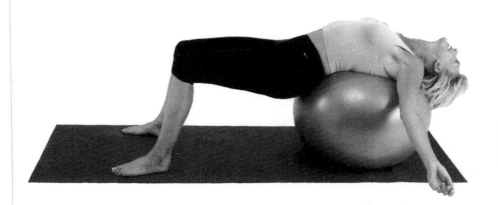

Front Raise, Standing

level: beginning–advanced

benefits: This targets the front shoulder muscles.

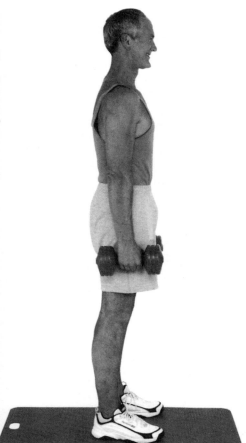

1 Stand with feet slightly apart, in good alignment, drawing your abdominal muscles in and up, and your shoulder blades in and down, away from the ears. Hold a weight at your sides, with the palms facing in toward your thighs. Inhale.

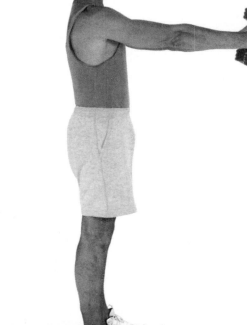

2 Exhale as you slowly raise the weights straight forward, to just below shoulder height. Pause, then slowly lower as you inhale. Repeat 10–15 times. Rest, and repeat the set once or twice more.

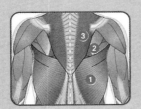

Side of Back Muscles (❶ Latissimus Dorsi), Upper and Mid-Back Muscles (❷ Rhomboids and ❸ Mid- Trapezius) These muscles strengthen the upper body core by pulling the shoulders down and retracting the shoulder blades toward the spine. This protects the shoulders from injury resulting from poor upper back alignment.

The Woodchopper   level: beginning–advanced

benefits: Strengthens the side and mid-back muscles as well as the muscles that allow you to draw the shoulder blades in and down, to build a stabilizing upper body core.

tips: This is a good transitional exercise to do between working the front of the chest/shoulders and the upper back. ▬ It feels especially good if you have tense shoulders from hunching over a computer or worktable. It provides a wonderful stretch to the entire upper body, especially if you are vigilant about keeping your lower back from arching as you lower the weights. ▬ Keep those shoulders down, for the best stretch as you strengthen.

1 Lie on the floor with both knees bent and the feet flat. Holding a weight in each hand, palms facing each other, press the weights up above the center of your chest, drawing your shoulders down away from your ears and in toward each other. Slightly round your elbows, and keep them rounded this way throughout the exercise. Pull your abdomen in and up. Inhale.

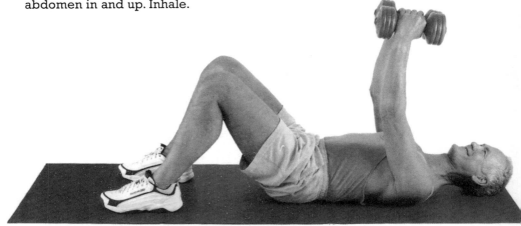

2 Exhale as you slowly lower the weights toward the floor above your head, without arching the lower back or hunching the shoulders. (Stop lowering the weights if either begins to occur.)

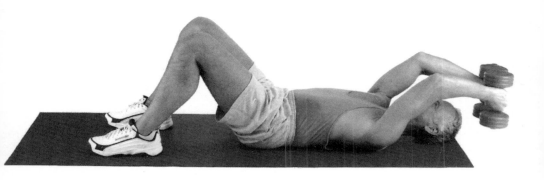

3 Continue to exhale as you pull the weights back up to just above your chest, bending your elbows as you do so. Pause and inhale, then repeat. Repeat 10–15 times. Rest, and repeat once more.

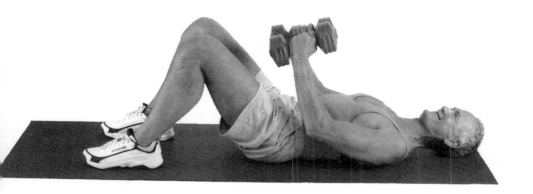

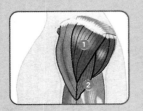

Arm Lift Muscles (❶ Medial Deltoids and ❷ Posterior Deltoids) The medial, or middle, deltoids lift the arms to the side and give the shoulders a nice shape. The posterior, or rear, deltoids move your arms backward and help to hold the upper arm in correct alignment.

Reverse Fly   level: beginning–advanced

benefits: Strengthens the upper and mid-back and the back of the shoulders.

tips: Pause for a second at the height of the lift as you consciously complete your exhale. This will strengthen your core and support your back. ▪ If this exercise feels too challenging, work up to it by practicing the following One-Arm Row (page 90).

1 Stand with the feet hip-width apart and the knees slightly bent. Hold a weight in each hand beneath your shoulders with your palms facing each other and elbows slightly rounded. Hinge forward from the hips, lifting the abdominals in and up and pulling the shoulder blades in and down to keep your back safely aligned. Look at a spot on the floor about 5 feet (1.5 m) in front of you to position your head correctly. Inhale.

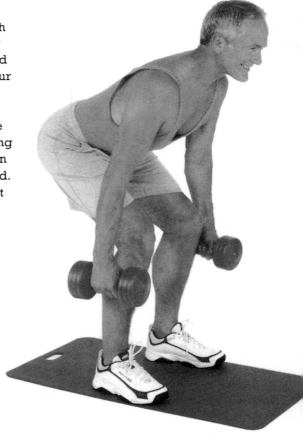

2 Exhale as you raise your arms until the weights are nearly level with your shoulders, elbows pointing up. Feel the strengthening squeeze between the shoulder blades. Slowly lower the weights to return. Repeat 10–15 times. Rest and repeat the set once or twice.

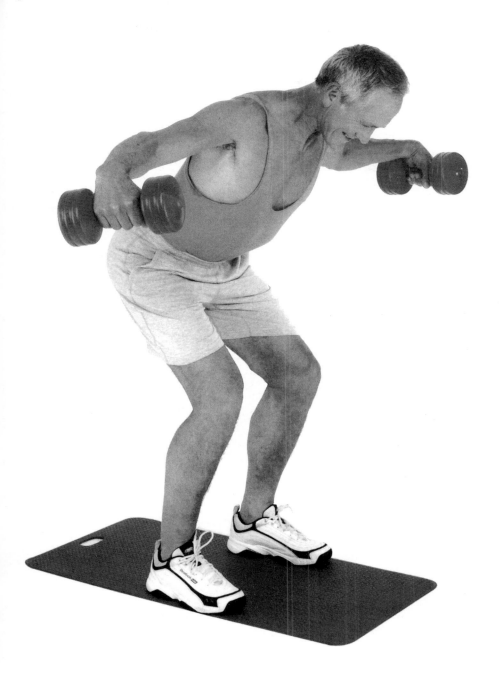

One-Arm Row   level: beginning–advanced

benefits: Strengthens the mid-back, sides of the back, and the rear shoulders.

tips: Try to keep the working arm close to your body as it lifts and lowers the weight, as if you were gently scraping it against your side ribs. This will help target the correct muscles. ■ Keep the shoulders and hips parallel to each other by keeping both sides of the waist long.

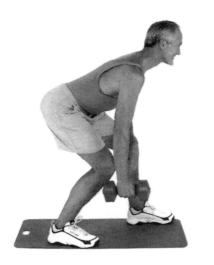

1 Stand with the feet hip-width apart, holding a weight in the right hand and letting it hang straight down below the right shoulder with the palm facing the thigh. Strongly pull the shoulders down and in toward each other. Take a large step with the left foot, bending your knees as you do so. Rest your left elbow or forearm on top of the left knee for support. Inhale.

2 Exhale as you pull the weight up toward the right hip, squeezing the shoulder blades firmly in and down. The right elbow should point up toward the ceiling. Inhale and lower the weight without rounding that right shoulder forward. Repeat 10–15 times, then change sides. Rest, then repeat the set.

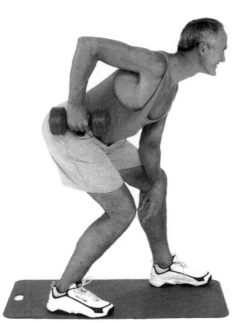

Variation

Instead of resting your forearm on your forward thigh, cross it behind your lower back. This strengthens the back muscles.

Pull-Across Stretch for Shoulders

benefits: Stretches the mid-/upper back and the back of the shoulders.

Hold your left arm out to the side, then fold it across your chest, with the thumb facing up. Use your right hand to gently pull the left arm toward your chest until you feel a stretch in the middle of your back and/or behind your left shoulder. Hold for a few breaths, then change sides.

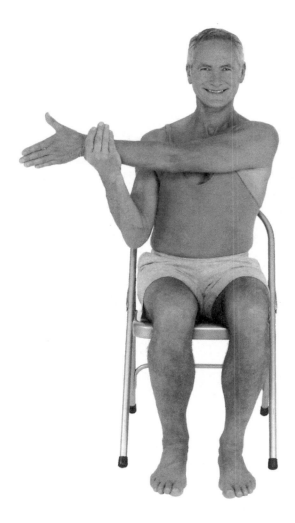

Lateral Raise   level: beginning–advanced

benefits: Strengthens the middle of the top of the shoulder along with the front and back shoulder muscles.

tips: This is a classic "shaper-upper" for the shoulders. ■ It can be advanced by gradually working up to lifting heavier weights.

1 Stand with the feet hip-width apart, abdominals in and up, and shoulder blades down and in toward each other. The knees should be slightly bent. Hold a weight in each hand, palms facing forward and upper arms rotated outward. Inhale.

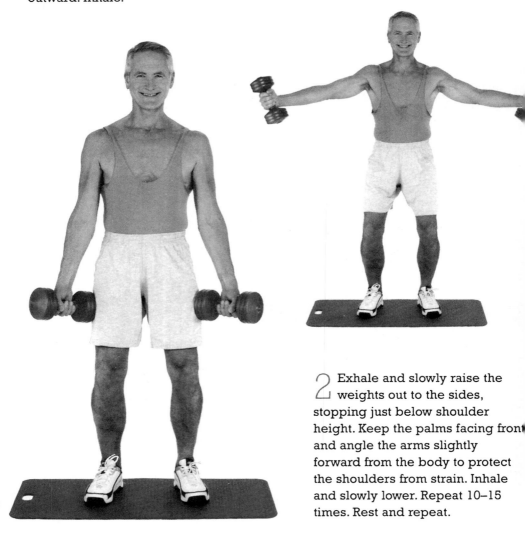

2 Exhale and slowly raise the weights out to the sides, stopping just below shoulder height. Keep the palms facing front and angle the arms slightly forward from the body to protect the shoulders from strain. Inhale and slowly lower. Repeat 10–15 times. Rest and repeat.

Head Tilt with Clasped Hands

benefits: Stretches the sides of the neck and the tops of the shoulders. Use this stretch throughout your workout, whenever you need a little break.

tips: "Less is more" with this and nearly all neck stretches. Even a small tilt may create a very big stretch ! ▬ Remember the Up against the Wall exercise (page 35)? Keep the lower core muscles pulled in and up as you do the Head Tilt so that your lower back doesn't arch into an excessive, spine-stressing curve.

❶ Stand in correct alignment, feet slightly apart, then roll the shoulders back and in, clasping your hands together behind you to make one fist; this will "lock" the shoulders into their retracted position. Pull the shoulders down away from your ears, as much as you can. Your arms should be close to your body.

❷ Maintain this position and keep the shoulders level as you tilt your head to one side until you feel a stretch. Hold and breathe 4–6 deep, slow breaths. Return your head to the upright position, then stretch to the other side.

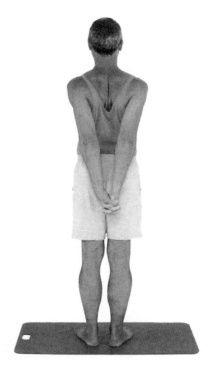
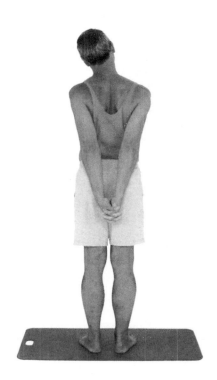

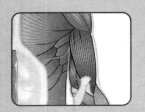

Front Upper Arm Muscles (Biceps) These are the muscles that allow the arm to flex, or bend, at the elbow. They also provide lifting and pulling strength.

Biceps Curl   level: beginning–advanced

benefits: Strengthens the muscles in the front of the upper arm.

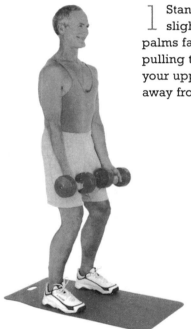

1 Stand with your feet hip-width apart and your knees slightly bent, holding a weight in each hand, with the palms facing forward. Strongly engage your lower core by pulling the abdominals in and the pelvic floor up. Engage your upper core by drawing the shoulders in and down, away from the ears.

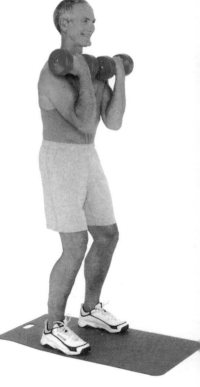

2 Exhale, and slowly "curl" the weights up to the front of your shoulders, squeezing your forearms against your upper arms as if you were crushing a grape. Inhale as you slowly lower the weights. Repeat 10–15 times. Rest and repeat the set once or twice more.

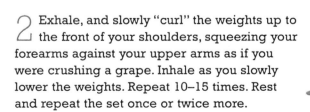

Hammer Curl   level: beginning–advanced

benefits: Strengthens the "long head" of this two-part muscle.

tips: A nice way to work the biceps is to alternate between one set of biceps curls and one set of hammer curls.

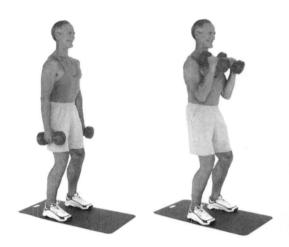

1 Stand with your feet hip-width apart and your knees slightly bent, holding a weight in each hand, with the palms facing in toward each other, the way you would hold a hammer. Inhale.

2 Exhale, and slowly "curl" the weights up to the front of your shoulders, squeezing your forearms against your upper arms. Inhale as you slowly lower the weights. The palms will face each other the entire time. Repeat 10–15 times. Rest and repeat the set once or twice more.

FOLLOW-UP STRETCH

The "So Big Stretch"

benefits: Relaxes and lengthens the biceps muscles.

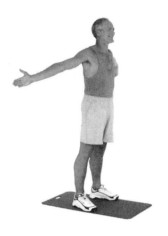

❶ Stand in good alignment with feet slightly apart. Keeping your core muscles engaged so that your back doesn't arch, open your arms straight out to the sides with the palms flexed and the fingers pointing back. Inhale deeply, moving arms further back to increase the stretch, if you'd like.

❷ Exhale, letting the shoulders drop if they've begun to creep up toward your ears. Inhale and repeat, moving the arms even further back if you can, then lower the arms and rest. Repeat as many times as you'd like.

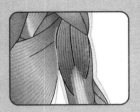

Back Upper Arm Muscles (Triceps) These muscles straighten the elbow (extension) and provide pushing strength. They are usually of marked interest to the over-50 woman, as they eliminate upper arm jiggle when they are strong and toned.

Kickbacks, Standing

level: beginning–advanced

benefits: Strengthens the muscles on the back of the upper arms as well as the upper and mid-back muscles.

tips: Keep your upper arms tight against your torso for maximum muscular engagement. ▬ If this feels too strenuous, try working one arm at a time until you get stronger. Rest the hand of the non-working arm on the top of your thigh to help your shoulders stay "squared."

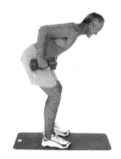

1 Stand with your feet hip-width apart and your knees bent. Hold a weight in each hand, palms facing the sides of your thighs. Engage your core muscles as you tilt forward from your hips until your body is at about a 45-degree angle to the floor. Bend your elbows, pointing them back and up behind you. Draw the shoulders firmly down, away from your ears and in toward each other. (This by itself is a great exercise for the upper back!) Inhale, keeping the eyes directed to a spot about 4 feet (1.2 m) ahead, on the floor.

2 Exhale as you slowly press the weights up behind you, straightening the arms without lowering them. Hold for a beat, then slowly bend the elbows, bringing the weights back to the starting position. Repeat 10–15 times. Rest and repeat the set once or twice more.

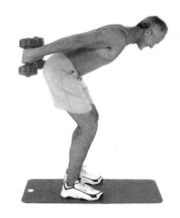

Triceps Extensions, Supine

level: beginning–advanced

benefits: Provides an alternative way to strengthen the triceps, one that doesn't stress the back. This may make it easier for you to try using heavier weights, for further challenge.

tips: If you wish, you can support the arm that's holding the weight by grasping it just below the elbow with your other hand.

1 Lie on the floor, with both knees bent and the feet flat. Hold a weight in your right hand, and press it straight up so it is directly above your right shoulder. The palm should face left. Pull the shoulders down away from the ears, and engage your lower core muscles. Inhale.

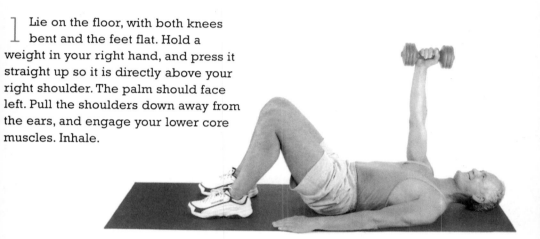

2 Exhale as you very slowly bend the right elbow to 90 degrees, without allowing the elbow to change its position in space. Move the weight in the direction of the floor behind you. Inhale as you slowly press the weight back up to the starting position. Repeat 10–15 times. Rest and repeat using the other arm.

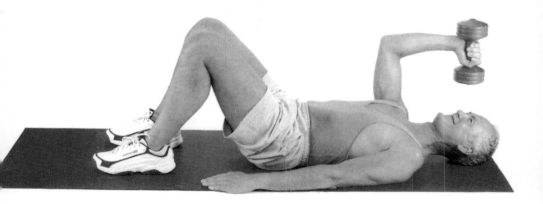

Triceps Dips   level: intermediate–advanced

benefits: This excellent triceps strengthener can be done with no equipment at all. It is a very challenging exercise, requiring close attention to upper back alignment. If you apply your upper core stabilizing skills, you will master the triceps dips quickly and be pleased by the results they bring.

1 Sit on the edge of a sturdy chair with nonslip feet, or a bench, with your hands next to you and fingers curled forward over the edge of the support. Place your feet flat on the floor, slightly ahead of your knees, with your toes facing forward. Bring your arms tight against your body then slide your bottom off until your arms are holding most of your weight. Press the shoulders down firmly, and keep them down throughout.

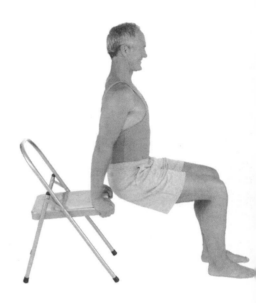

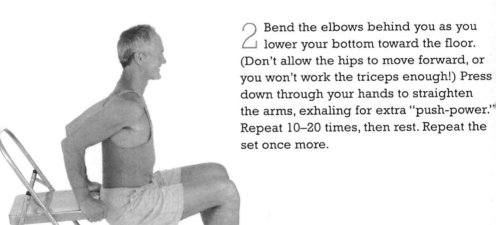

2 Bend the elbows behind you as you lower your bottom toward the floor. (Don't allow the hips to move forward, or you won't work the triceps enough!) Press down through your hands to straighten the arms, exhaling for extra "push-power." Repeat 10–20 times, then rest. Repeat the set once more.

Scratch Your Back Stretch

benefits: This gives the triceps muscles a good stretch. It also greatly increases shoulder mobility.

tips: Men, who tend to be more muscular in their upper bodies, may find this stretch to be especially challenging. This means, of course, they really need to do it! ■ This stretch can also be done standing.

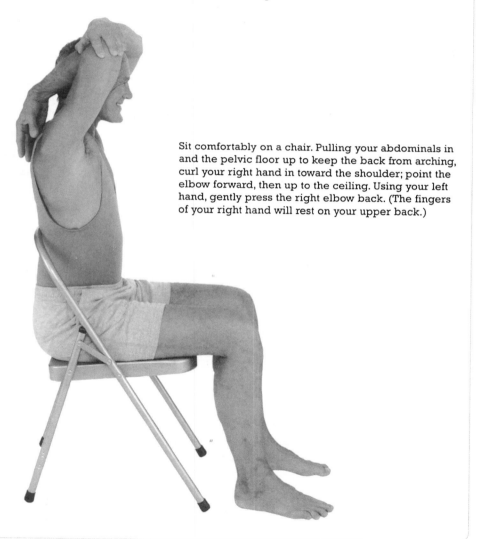

Sit comfortably on a chair. Pulling your abdominals in and the pelvic floor up to keep the back from arching, curl your right hand in toward the shoulder; point the elbow forward, then up to the ceiling. Using your left hand, gently press the right elbow back. (The fingers of your right hand will rest on your upper back.)

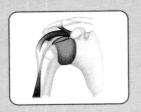

Upper Arm/Shoulder Blade Attaching Muscles (Rotator Cuff) The rotator cuff muscles attach the upper arm bones to the shoulder blades. They allow the arms a full 360 degrees of mobility and help stabilize the shoulder joint. Good upper back alignment will help prevent injury to this muscle group.

Drawbridge for External Rotators

level: beginning–advanced

benefits: Strengthens the muscles that turn the upper arm out, away from the center of your chest. This action supports correct upper body alignment and helps prevent shoulder injuries.

tips: Keep the shoulder blades drawn in and down away from the ears. ■ Keep the lower back stabilized by activating your core abdominal strength.

1 Lie on your left side, with both knees bent in front of you. Rest your head on the left arm, or on a small pillow, so your neck is comfortable and your head is aligned with your shoulders and hips. Hold a light weight in the right hand, knuckles down, and with the right elbow bent to 90 degrees. Keep the elbow pressed firmly against the top of your waist throughout.

2 Slowly raise the weight to vertical, pivoting around the stationary elbow. Slowly lower the weight back to the floor. Repeat 10–15 times, then rest. Repeat on the opposite side, then do another set or two, alternating sides.

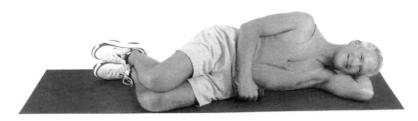

The Boat   level: intermediate–advanced

benefits: This will strengthen a healthy back even more.

tips: This should feel challenging, but not strenuous. Keep the legs low at first, if your lower back feels stressed. You will still get the strengthening benefits. ■ Think of this as a breathing exercise. Yes, your back muscles are working hard, but by focusing on taking deep, relaxed breaths, you will create a long, flexible and strong spine. You will also draw nourishing oxygen deep into your body's muscles and tissues.

1 Lie face down, resting your forehead on a folded towel. Rest your arms on the floor next to your body, with the backs of the hands on the floor. Draw your shoulders down, away from your ears. Strongly engage your lower core and actively extend the legs backward, with all 10 toenails facing the floor.

2 Maintaining your core support, raise your legs off the floor, along with your head, chest, and shoulders. (Your hands remain on the floor.) Look about 3 feet (90 cm) in front of you keeping your neck long and strain-free. Hold and breathe deeply for three or four breaths, then lower the legs and upper body and relax completely, head to one side. Enjoy the energizing effect on the body. Repeat twice more.

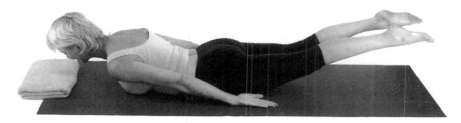

Variation

If you are strong enough, you may also raise your arms to give the front of the body a good stretch.

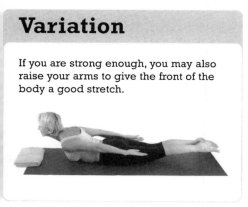

FOLLOW-UP STRETCH

Child's Pose

(page 28)

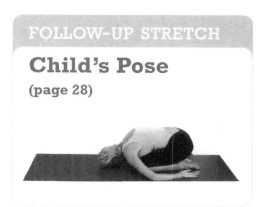

Correct Sitting, Lifting, and Carrying

The way you align your back can either make you stronger or lead to many strains and injuries, some quite serious. Whether bending over to lift an object, carrying something heavy, or simply sitting in a chair, you must maintain your lumbar, or lower back curve to protect your back and provide you with maximum functional strength.

Sitting deserves a careful look. We spend a lot of time sitting and frankly, most of us do it wrong. The problem is worsened by the fact that most chairs are poorly designed. Sitting slumped over a computer or desk for hours can lead to all sorts of spinal problems.

Correct Lifting Technique

benefits: Protects your back from strain and injury, by training the muscles to stabilize the spine in neutral alignment as you lift weight.

Tilt forward from your hips. Keep your shoulder blades pulled down and away from your ears, and in toward each other. Engage your abdominals, and create a "duck tail" by sticking your butt out. This will secure your lower spine into a strong, neutral curve. Bend your knees, placing one foot as far ahead of the other as is practical. Get as close to the object you are about to lift as you can. Hold it in to your body as you straighten the legs and lift.

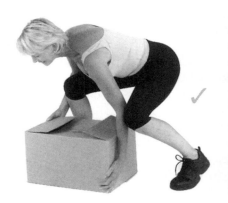

Incorrect Lifting Technique

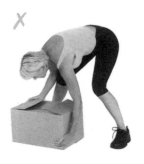

If you fail to maintain the neutral ("duck tail") curve in your lower back as you lift, you subject your spine to tremendous, possibly dangerous, stress. "Lifting with the legs" is not enough! And if you cannot get close enough to the object (for example, reaching for something in the back of a closet), don't lift it!

One more crucial precaution: never twist the body while lifting an object. It you do, you risk injuring your intervertebral discs.

Correct Carrying Technique

benefits: Protects your back from injury and strain by incorporating correct alignment and core support.

Always hold heavy objects close to your body. Maintain strong abdominal core support to protect your lumbar curve. Keep your shoulder blades pulled in toward each other so that the weight you are carrying can't pull your spine forward into an injury-risking slouch. You may be surprised at how much stronger this will allow you to be.

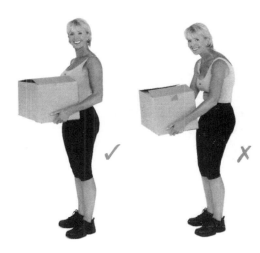

Seated Posture

benefits: Corrects posture, so that faulty alignment doesn't cause back pain and injury. Strengthens the muscular habits that support this healthy alignment.

When we are standing, our weight is balanced over our two feet. When we are sitting, our "sit bones"—the two bones on the bottom of the pelvis that you feel if you are sitting on a hard bench—are our "feet." Try to balance directly on top of those two bones. If you tuck your tail you will feel yourself rolling to the back of the sit-bones, thus flattening out the lumbar curve. Try rocking your pelvis forward and back a little, until you sense that you are sitting right on top of your sit bones. You will notice a slight forward curve in your lower back. That lumbar curve is the healthiest, strongest position for your lower back. In fact, over the years, I have come to refer to it as the "strong back curve."

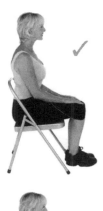

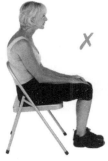

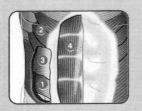

Abdominal Muscles (❶ Transverse Abdominus, ❷ External Obliques, ❸ Internal Obliques, and ❹ Rectus Abdominus) These muscles bend, rotate, and support the spine. They balance the back muscles in providin core support, strength, and mobility to your body. Work them correctly and your reward will be a nice, tight waistline.

Table 1   level: beginning

benefits: Strengthens all layers of the abdominal muscles by training them to pull in and up as they contract. This reinforces core strength and also helps to flatten the profile of your stomach! This exercise is safe to do if you have osteoporosis.

tips: If your lower back arches or registers any strain, try not moving your thighs so far away from your chest at first. ▬ Are your shoulder and neck muscles getting into the act by tensing up? If they are, consciously relax them; they are mistakenly doing the stabilizing work that your abdominals should be doing.

1 Lie on your back with both knees folded in toward your chest and your arms by your sides. Exhale as you engage the deep abdominal core, pulling the abdominal muscles in and up, and lifting the floor of the pelvis.

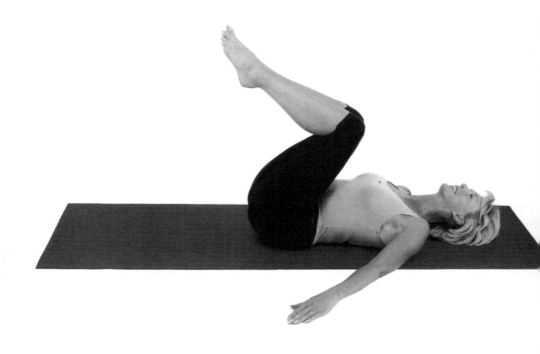

2 Maintain this core support as you move the knees forward to a vertical position above the hips, making a 90-degree angle. Your shins will be parallel to the floor and each other. Check to see that your core muscles are still strongly engaged, and that your lower back hasn't arched up. Hold this position for three breaths, then fold the knees back in toward the chest and rest. Breathe normally for a moment, and then repeat. Repeat for a total of 5–10 times.

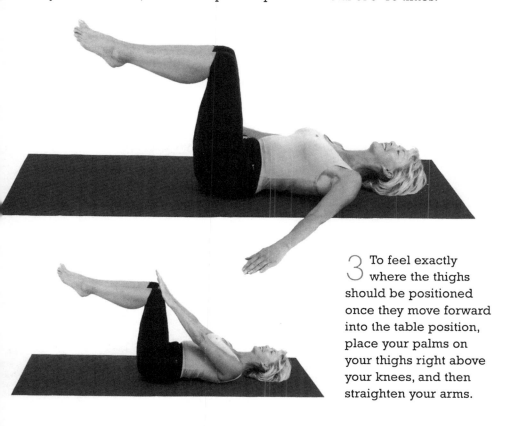

3 To feel exactly where the thighs should be positioned once they move forward into the table position, place your palms on your thighs right above your knees, and then straighten your arms.

Variation

If you feel lower back strain, do the Table one leg at a time: hold one leg in the folded-in position as the other moves forward.

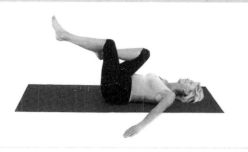

Table 2   level: beginning–intermediate

benefits: Further strengthens the abdominal core without straining the back. Like Table 1, this exercise is safe to do if you have osteoporosis.

tips: If your lower back arches up, try pulling the abs in more strongly. ■ If the back still arches up or feels strained, don't lower your heel so close to the floor; even if you can only manage 2 inches (5 cm), you will still receive the benefits of this exercise. ■ Your breathing should reflect your effort. Exhale strongly, even audibly, when you need help in pulling the abdominals in toward your spine. Inhale into your upper lungs and sides of your body and back. In this way you will be able to draw adequate oxygen into the body without sacrificing your core support.

1 Lie on your back with both knees folded in toward your chest and your arms by your sides. Exhale as you engage the deep abdominal core and lift the floor of the pelvis. Maintain this core support as you move the knees forward to a vertical position above the hips, making a 90-degree angle. Your shins will be parallel to the floor and each other. Relax your shoulders!

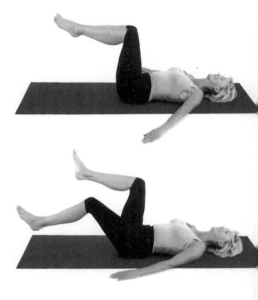

2 Keep your right knee exactly where it is as you lower your left heel toward the floor, maintaining the 90-degree angle at the back of the left knee. Make sure your lower back doesn't arch up.

3 Return the left knee to its vertical starting position. Repeat, lowering the right heel while keeping the left knee in place above your left hip. Do 8–10 repetitions, alternating sides, then rest.

FOLLOW-UP STRETCH

Spiral Stretch
(page 76)

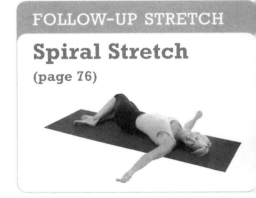

Oblique Curl-Up   level: beginning–advanced

benefits: Strengthens all layers of the abdominal muscles, especially the external and internal obliques. These are the muscles most important for supporting the back. The obliques also do more to flatten the stomach than the much smaller, "six pack" rectus abdominus!

tips: This exercise is **not** recommended if you have osteoporosis. Learn to keep your neck relaxed as you lift and twist from the waist. In essence your head is the weight that your abdominals are lifting. If you pull the head forward with your hands, this strengthening won't be able to occur and you may hurt your neck. Once you understand how to do this correctly and consistently, then you are ready to move on to the Bicycle Crunch (page 112).

1 Lie on your back with your knees bent and your feet flat on the floor. Place your hands behind your head, and relax the weight of your head into your palms. Raise your left leg until it is perpendicular to the floor; the left knee may be bent. Inhale.

2 Exhale, curving your upper spine up until both shoulder blades leave the floor. Do not pull on your head! Use your abs to lift a little higher and twist at the waist, until your chest faces the left leg. Try to keep the elbows open to the sides, in line with your ears, as you twist. Lower the body and inhale. Repeat 10–20 times to one side, and then place both feet on the floor and rest for a moment.

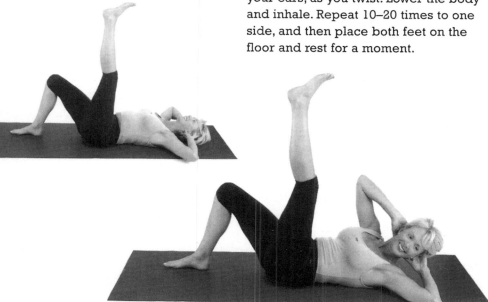

3 Rotate your head gently side-to-side to relax the neck muscles, which may have tightened up, then repeat to the other side.

Bicycle Crunch   level: intermediate–advanced

benefits: Recent research shows that this exercise is 300 percent more effective than the classic crunch! Along with working the rectus abdominus, it targets the external obliques, the muscles that do the most to create a firm, trim waistline.

tips: This exercise is **not** recommended if you have osteoporosis. Exhale sharply each time the knee comes in, taking a quick inhale as you switch sides. ▬ Keep elbows open as you twist. If you allow the top elbow to cross over your face as you twist, chances are you will be pulling on your head and using your shoulders, not your waistline muscles, to do the work. This puts an enormous amount of strain on the neck and won't give you that 300 percent more benefit.

1 Lie on your back with your hands beneath your head and both knees drawn into your chest. Pull your abdominals in and up and lift the floor of the pelvis to engage your lower core. Draw the shoulders down, away from your ears. Inhale.

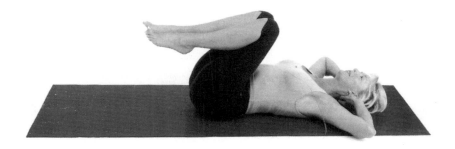

2 Exhale, curving your upper spine up until both shoulder blades leave the floor. At the same time, bring your left knee in toward your chest, and twist at the waist, bringing your right elbow toward the left knee. Extend the right leg up, anywhere from 45 degrees to a full 90 degrees above the floor.

3 Switch sides, simultaneously twisting to the right as the right knee comes in and the left leg straightens. Keep your upper body curved up, away from the floor. Repeat 20 times, alternating sides, then rest. Repeat the set.

Spiral Stretch

(page 76)

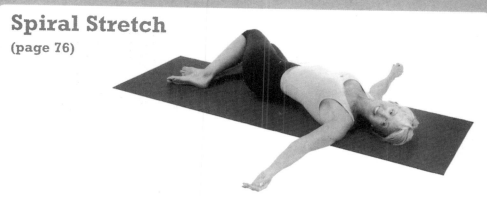

Standing Side Stretch

benefits: A simple way to stretch the obliques as well as the deep muscles on the sides of your lower back.

tips: Place your nonreaching hand flat on the side of the thigh for added support and stability.

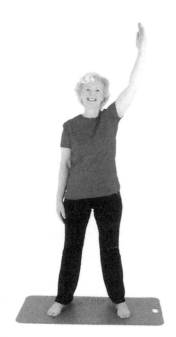

❶ Stand with your feet about shoulder-width apart and your back in neutral alignment. Engage the lower core muscles by pulling the abs in and up, and lifting the pelvic floor. Raise your left arm to vertical, with the palm facing right. Inhale, stretching your ribs up, away from the hips.

❷ Keep this feeling of length in both sides of your body as you reach the left arm up and over toward the right, until you feel a stretch. Stay here and breathe for three or four breaths, then return to vertical and lower the arm to rest. Repeat on the other side.

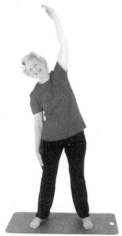

Stability Ball Curl-Up

level: intermediate–advanced

benefits: Like the Bicycle Crunch, this exercise has been shown to recruit more abdominal muscle than the traditional crunch. By using a large stability ball, the core muscles will do additional work as they help you maintain balance.

tips: Be sure your bottom doesn't roll forward, off the ball. If this happens you will be working your legs, more than your abs.

1 Sit on the floor with a large stability ball against your lower back, stabilizing the ball between your hands.

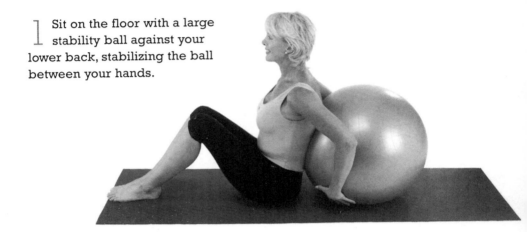

2 Slowly roll backward onto the ball, until your entire spine is supported by it, from your head to your tail. Pause here, making sure you are safely and comfortably balanced (this should feel great!). Place your hands behind your head, keeping your neck long and relaxed. Your feet should be hip-width apart, parallel to each other, and planted firmly on the floor. Inhale.

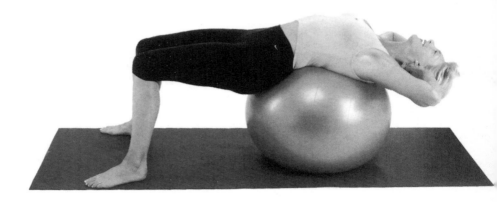

3 As you exhale, slowly curl your upper back up off the ball and twist to the left. Be sure to use your abdominals to accomplish this: don't pull on your head! Slowly lower back down to the ball as you inhale. Repeat, alternating sides, 20–30 times.

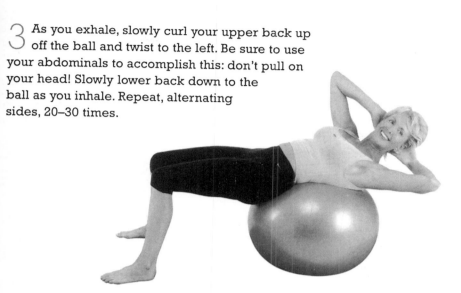

FOLLOW-UP STRETCH

Supine Chest Stretch
(page 49)

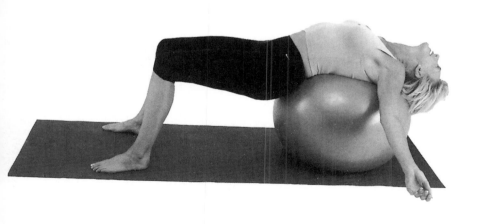

Putting it all Together

The yoga-based Plank is a near-perfect upper and lower body core strengthener. It is also a great way to strengthen your shoulders, upper back, arms, and legs. The Plank will give you a concrete sense of how to work the front of the body and the back of the body together, as a powerful unit. Many trainers use it for this reason, since it teaches you how to use your abdominals to support the back in an unmistakable way.

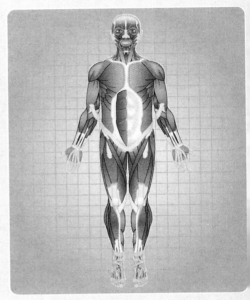

The Plank provides you with an opportunity to practice deep, steady breathing, too. By breathing in this mindful way as you perform such a challenging pose, you can learn to work hard, without accumulating excess tension of either the mental or physical variety.

The Plank is a good exercise to do on a daily basis. As you gain strength you will be able to hold the pose longer and longer. This is a good bench mark by which to measure your progress and is an excellent way to keep growing strong, centered, and energized.

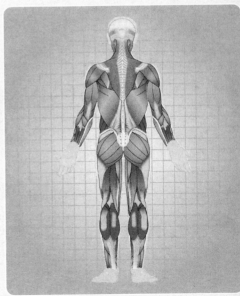

The Plank   level: beginning

benefits: One of the very best core strengtheners, and safe to do even if you have osteoporosis. "The Plank" also strengthens the shoulders, arms and chest muscles.

tips: Work up to holding the Plank for thirty, and then sixty seconds. You may be surprised how aerobic this seemingly motionless pose becomes! ▬ If this position is too challenging, place your knees on the floor, maintaining a straight line from your ears to your hips, as in "Knee Push-Ups", page 46. It will still be very effective.

1 Rest on your knees and forearms, with fingers facing forward and palms flat on the floor. Your elbows should be directly below your shoulders, your shoulders should be down, away from your ears, and your head should be in alignment with the spine. Make sure your neck is long and your nose is pointing toward the floor.

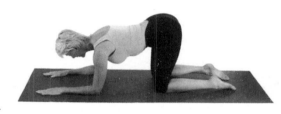

2 Strongly contract your abdominal muscles in and your pelvic floor muscles up, activating your lower core support as you reach the right leg straight back, tucking the toes under.

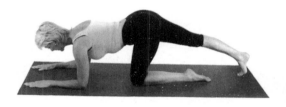

3 Reach the left leg straight back to join the right, again tucking the toes under. Firm your leg muscles to straighten the knees. Hold this position for at least three breaths, using your core support to prevent the back from sagging down toward the floor. Continue to reach the heels back, and remember to keep the shoulders pulled down and in, in order to widen the front of the chest.

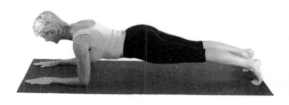

4 To return to the starting position, gently lower your knees to the floor, and then sit back into Child's Pose (page 28) to rest. Repeat three times, holding the pose for as long as you can.

Plank with Leg Raise

level: intermediate–advanced

benefits: This variation will strengthen the core muscles even more, as it gives the gluteals and hamstrings a workout, too.

1 Assume the basic Plank position (page 117, Step 3).

2 Keeping your core muscles strongly engaged, raise the right leg 1–2 feet (30–60 cm) off the floor. Hold this position for two or three breaths, then lower the leg to the starting position. Repeat with the other leg. Repeat 4 times, alternating legs.

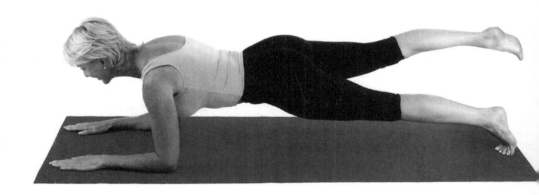

3 To return to the starting position, gently lower your knees to the floor, and then sit back into Child's Pose (page 28) to rest.

Side-Lying Plank

level: intermediate–advanced

benefits: Strengthens the shoulders, the upper and lower core muscles, the legs, and especially the external and internal obliques.

1 Lie on your right side, propped on the right forearm. Put the right elbow beneath the right shoulder, palm flat on the floor. Extend the right leg so head, shoulders, hips, and right ankle are in a straight line. Place the sole of the left foot on the floor in front of your right thigh, left knee toward the ceiling and left arm on left thigh.

2 Press down into your right forearm, palm, and left foot, raising the underneath hip off the floor. The outside of that right foot will still be on the floor. You will feel the waistline muscles working very hard, especially on the underneath side of your body. Stop here, if you are struggling with maintaining core support of your back.

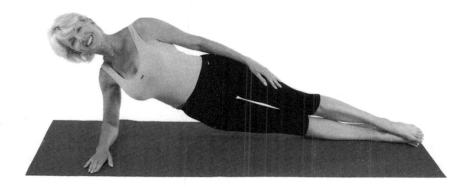

3 For the full pose, straighten your left leg, resting it on top of your right leg. Both knees and ankles should face straight ahead of you. Keep your body in one straight line. Hold for three or four breaths, then slowly lower the right hip to the floor and rest. Repeat twice more on this side, then change sides.

FOLLOW-UP STRETCH

Child's Pose
(page 28)

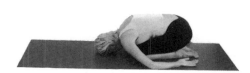

Cooling Down

The cool-down serves an important purpose, especially for older adults or those with any cardiovascular problems, as it allows the body to gradually slow down from a vigorous workout. In this way, the heart is not stressed by a sudden halt in activity. If you have worked up a sweat and are breathing heavily from your strengthening session, take the time to do some mild, nonstrenuous movements, such as walking around or gently stretching for a few minutes, until your breathing returns to normal. This will provide your cardiovascular system with a transitional period during which your heart rate can slowly return to normal. In essence, you are reversing the preparatory process you went through as you warmed up.

The cool-down should be something you look forward to. It is your reward, and an opportunity to enjoy the sensation of well-being that always accompanies a good, hard workout. Once your breathing and heart-rate are back to normal, treat yourself to a relaxing stretch. Take a moment to listen to your body. What is it asking for today? Any stretch that comes to mind/body is probably a good choice. There is nothing wrong with simply choosing the ones that feel best; chances are, those are the stretches your body needs most! Whatever stretches your muscles request, this is your opportunity to refresh them by taking deep, nourishing breaths. Maybe your lower back would appreciate a gentle stretch, such as the Rock and Roll (page 29), or maybe your neck feels like it could use a Head Tilt Stretch (page 93), followed by some casual shoulder rolls. Once you do that, perhaps a moment to do the Step Through the Door Stretch (page 48) is in order. You get the idea—improvise your stretching sequence, based on what you feel would be appropriate for you on that particular day. The cooling-down process should, ideally, take about 10 minutes or more.

Legs up the Wall Pose

benefits: This restorative pose will rest your cardiovascular system as it refreshes your entire body. By semi-inverting the body, it reverses the usual circulatory flow, giving the veins and arteries a rest as it floods the upper body with nourishing, oxygenated blood. (Note: Recent research shows that the blood supply to the brain diminishes over the years. The Legs up the Wall Pose reverses this.) This pose can also be used to gently stretch the hamstrings. Do the Legs up the Wall Pose at the very end of your workout, after your cool-down is complete.

tips: This is a superb way to relax and stretch a tight lower back. ▬ This is a good pose to do at any time. It feels great after a long day on your feet (it is what dancers do to rest during breaks in rehearsals), and is the perfect antidote to that sluggish feeling that follows long plane or car trips. ▬ If you prefer not to stretch your hamstrings, move your body back away from the wall until the sensation of stretch ceases.

1 Sit on the floor, with the side of your body near a wall. Roll onto your back, pulling your knees into your chest.

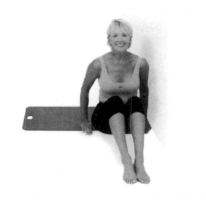

2 Rest your heels on the wall, taking your legs straight up; your knees should be fairly straight. If this creates too much pull in the back of your legs, simply squirm your bottom away from the wall, until the stretch in the back of your legs is comfortable. Rest your arms by your sides, palms up. Close your eyes. Focus your attention inward, following the breath as it slowly, automatically enters and then leaves your body. Allow your muscles to let go completely. Rest in this restorative pose for as long as you'd like. Try to stay in it for at least 5 minutes, in order to receive the benefits.

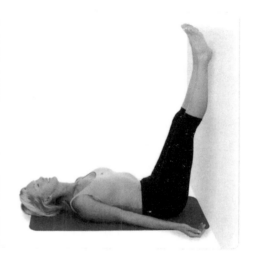

3 When you are finished, bend your knees and roll onto one side. Pause there for a breath or two, before slowly standing up.

Important note

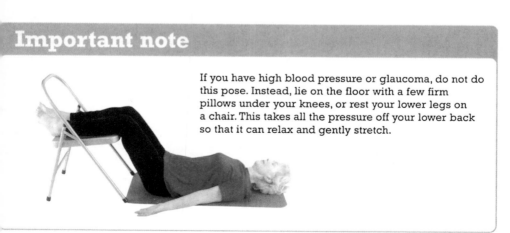

If you have high blood pressure or glaucoma, do not do this pose. Instead, lie on the floor with a few firm pillows under your knees, or rest your lower legs on a chair. This takes all the pressure off your lower back so that it can relax and gently stretch.

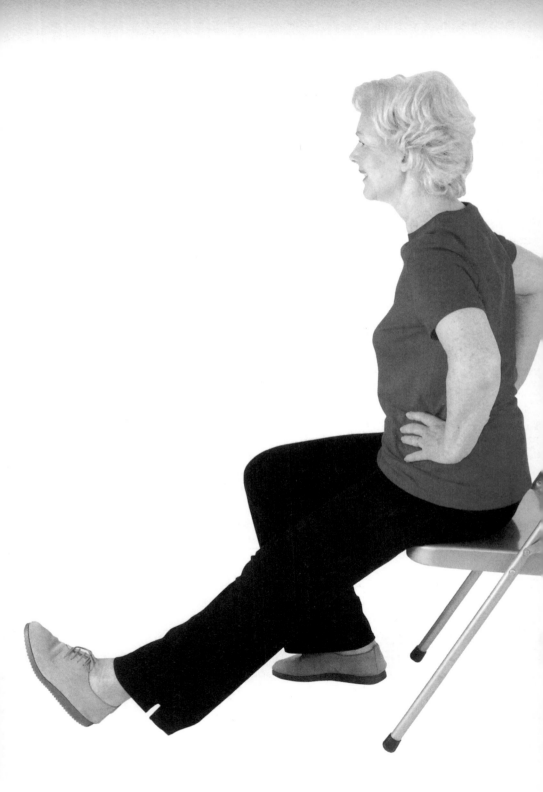

part 3   **special concerns**

> **balance**

> **arthritis**

> **osteoporosis**

> **strengthening for the out-of-shape over-65s**

> **chair exercises for strength**

> **chair exercises for flexibility**

Balance

No one likes to fall or stumble and as adults we have good reason to look closely at our balance skills; falling is no joke to weak or brittle bones, as anyone who has experienced a broken hip from a fall will attest. Perhaps because at times it seems so frustratingly beyond one's control, there is a common misconception that, as far as balance is concerned, "either you have it or you don't." In fact, balance skills can be improved. As a former ballet teacher of mine once said, "Balance isn't a gift of the holy ghost. You have to practice!"

We all have an inborn ability to remain upright or "catch" ourselves when surprised by a sudden shift in our footing. This doesn't require conscious attention; it just happens. As we grow older, however, this innate sense of balance begins to diminish. In part this has do to with changes in our vision, reflex speed, and the acuity of the nerve endings in our skin and joints that enable us to sense our position as we move. Compromised balance also results, however, from being generally deconditioned. Weak muscles cannot respond adequately when we find ourselves in unstable positions. Take an honest look at yourself. Have you grown more and more sedentary over the years? If so, your balance instincts have doubtlessly eroded, and could use a tune-up.

Postural changes occurring over time as we adjust to injuries or chronic pain, or develop bad habits such as slouching, also affect our balance. You may not be aware of these changes until one day you notice, perhaps, that walking on uneven surfaces or descending steep stairs has begun to feel awkward, even risky. Maybe your tennis or golf game has begun to suffer.

If you know that your muscles are weak from lack of exercise, one of the best things you can do to improve your balance is to commit to a general strengthening routine. For even better results, focus on the muscles that contribute the most to helping us "hold" our balance: the gluteus medius and the gluteus minimus, on the side and back of the hip. These are the "abductors" (see page 70). If you stand with your hands on your hips, then rotate your fingers backward and slightly down, you will be able to feel them. Now, as an experiment, shift your weight over one leg. Feel how the glutes on that side contract as soon as your weight shifts from two feet to one? That is precisely how these muscles help you remain upright and balanced, whether you are walking, running, or even just trying to put on a pair of pants while standing. Any and all of the Squat exercises described on pages 37–41 will be helpful toward strengthening the gluteus medius and the gluteus minimus, along with the larger gluteus maximus muscle (see page 53) and other muscles of the upper leg. To target these balance muscles more precisely, also be sure to regularly practice the abductor exercises on pages 70–75.

The other muscles that are important for maintaining balance are the muscles of the lower leg, ankle, and foot. Be sure to do the exercises for the gastrocnemius and foot dorsi flexors on pages 78–80 to build balance power from the ground up.

The following full-body exercises will help you feel, in an unmistakable way, how the abductors and the foot and ankle muscles hold your body in balance.

Corner Balance   level: beginning

benefits: Safely strengthens your sense of balance, in three simple steps.

tips: Don't worry if it is much harder for you to balance on one side than on the other. This is common. File the information away; it is part of your growing self-knowledge. In time, this exercise can help you regain symmetry in your balance skills. ■ Don't be disturbed by the wobbling actions that occur as you struggle to maintain your balance; those wobbles are the exercise. As you practice, you will strengthen your feet, your ankles and your hip muscles. In time, your balance confidence will grow stronger, too.

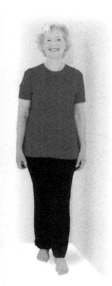

1 Stand in a corner, facing out. Position yourself so that your shoulders are about 3 inches (7 cm) away from the walls: in this way, you know that even if you lose your balance, you won't fall far or hurt yourself. Your back heel should be about 4–6 inches (10–15 cm) away from the corner. Place the other foot in front of the toes of the back foot, and slightly out to the side. Assume correct spinal alignment, engaging your lower core. Gaze straight ahead. Hold this position for 10 breaths, if you can.

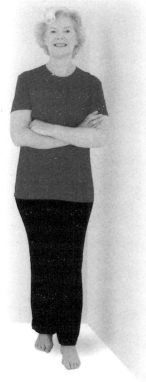

2 Now cross your arms in front of your chest. Be prepared—this small change makes it much more difficult to balance. Hold this position for 10 breaths, focusing straight ahead of you.

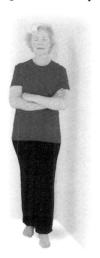

3 If you feel secure, then try closing your eyes. This is surprisingly difficult the first time. Just remember, the walls are there if you need them.

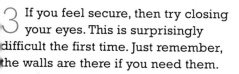

4 Repeat the three phases with the opposite foot in front.

Shifting the Weight from Foot to Foot

level: beginning–intermediate

benefits: Teaches and strengthens the weight-shifting skills that are the essence of balance in motion.

tips: Take your time when learning balancing skills. Enjoy noticing the little adjustments your body is learning to make. Pay attention to the very interesting relationship between your alignment, breathing, focus, and concentration.

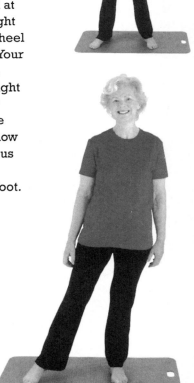

1 Stand with your feet slightly wider than hip-width apart and bring your back into neutral alignment. Engage your core. Relax your shoulders down away from your ears and draw them slightly in toward each other. Take a deep breath or two to help focus your concentration.

2 Shift your center of gravity (roughly located at your belly button), to the left, until it is straight above the center of the left ankle. The toes and heel of the left foot should be pressed into the floor. Your head should also be directly over the left ankle. Some of your weight will have shifted off your right foot, but you may leave that foot on the floor for balance. Check that your shoulders and hips are level. Pause here for at least 4 breaths, feeling how the muscles of your left leg, especially the gluteus medius muscles on the side of the hip, are contracting to stabilize your body over the left foot.

3 Shift your weight back onto both feet and rest for a moment, before shifting your weight over the right foot.

4 Continue to shift slowly from one foot to the other. Once your balance feels strong and secure try releasing the non-weight-bearing foot off the floor completely.

Tree Pose   level: intermediate–advanced

benefits: This challenging, one-legged pose from yoga will help you practice and strengthen your balance skills at a more advanced level.

tips: Once you feel balanced over one foot, firm the muscles of your standing leg, using them to "hug" the bones. This will help you hold that balance. ■ For an additional challenge, try reaching both arms up, above your shoulders, with the palms facing each other. Keep the shoulders pulled down away from your ears.

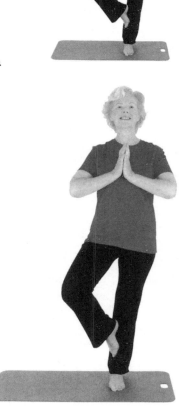

1 Stand in neutral alignment, engaging your core support by lifting the abdominals in and the pelvic floor up. Relax both shoulders down, away from your ears. Shift your weight over your left foot. Place the sole of your right foot against the inside of your left leg, either above or below the knee, which ever feels doable. Your hips and shoulders should be level. Hold your arms straight out to the sides, like a tightrope walker. Point your right knee to the side as much as possible without causing the hips to twist. Find a point straight ahead of you at eye level, and steadily focus your gaze on it. Breathe. Relax all extraneous muscular work.

2 Once you feel securely balanced, bend your elbows and place your palms against one another, in front of your chest. Draw your shoulders back and down, opening the chest. Breathe for 6–8 deep, slow breaths. Return the right foot to the floor and rest for a moment, before repeating on the other side.

Arthritis

Arthritis is a general term for a wide variety of conditions, all of which lead to pain or stiffness in the joints. It is estimated that around 40 million Americans suffer from either osteoarthritis or rheumatoid arthritis, the two most common forms. While there are different types of arthritis, medical authorities are in agreement on one point: if you have it, the most important thing for you to do is to keep moving.

Osteoarthritis occurs when the cartilage that covers the ends of the bones and serves as a shock absorber to the joints breaks down. There usually isn't much inflammation, but as the cartilage breaks down, pain occurs as the unprotected bones rub against one another.

Rheumatoid arthritis does cause inflammation. It affects the synovial tissue that lines the joint capsule, and can lead to deformation of the joint itself as other connective tissues become damaged. It can strike at any time, but usually occurs between the ages of 25 and 60.

Many people believe the pain of arthritis is a reason to exercise less, that this will protect their joints from further damage. In truth, that is the worst choice you could make. It is extremely important to keep exercising, no matter how severely affected you are. Strength training in particular is absolutely essential, as it takes the stress off affected joints by building up the surrounding muscles. Gentle, consistent stretching is also important, to preserve your range of movement.

On those bad days, when your joints are really hurting, go easy on your exercises. Take whatever antiinflammatory or pain reducer your doctor suggests. They won't cure the problem, but they will help you feel better, and if you aren't hurting you are more likely to do the exercises that will make you feel better, both immediately and long-term. Sometimes all it takes is 10 minutes with a heating pad to help get the circulation going and relieve the ache, or use inflammation-reducing ice. The choice is yours. Just keep moving!

Unfortunately, there is no cure for arthritis but you can protect your joints and keep symptoms from worsening.

■ **Commit to exercising at least several times a week.** Be moderate but consistent in your strength training, and stretch gently and often to maintain your range of motion.

■ **Keep your weight reasonable.** Every extra pound of weight places four times the stress on arthritic knees, hips, and feet when you walk or run.

■ **Make sure your posture is impeccable.** Poorly aligned bones are subject to wear and tear. Correct alignment will enable you to use your muscles better, build strength, and maintain a functional range of movement.

■ **Avoid repetitive strain.** Avoid over-doing extreme or high-impact activities. (There is a reason why football players and ballet dancers retire early, but swimmers and yogis go on forever.)

■ **Get enough rest.** People with arthritis say that fatigue, not pain, is their biggest complaint. The good news is, once you begin exercising, you will have more energy and may even sleep better, too.

Osteoporosis

Bones are not immutable; the body constantly loses and rebuilds bone cells. Osteoporosis occurs when bone loss occurs faster than manufacture. It is caused by diet, lack of exercise, or other factors. With osteoporosis, the bone's structure then becomes weak, sometimes leading to fractures. Often, osteoporosis is not diagnosed until a break occurs, but it is better to avoid the condition in the first place. Women over 65 and men over 70 should be sure to have a bone scan. (Men are susceptible to this disease, but it tends to occur later in their lives.)

Exercise helps your bones stay strong. It stimulates new bone growth, slows bone loss, and improves balance. Strength training 2–3 times a week along with 30–60 minutes of weight-bearing exercise such as walking on most days is usually adequate. By strengthening the back muscles and correcting poor alignment, you can avoid "dowager's hump" and prevent the almost undetectable spinal fractures that can gradually erode your vertebral structure.

A healthy diet, supplements of calcium, vitamin D, and magnesium can help with osteoporosis. Check with your doctor.

Strengthening for the Out-of-Shape over-65s

We all age at different rates. A fit, healthy 75-year-old will be able to do more and function better than a sedentary person of 60. Because of this, gerontologists use the term "functional age" as a truer measure of one's age. Recent, extensive studies confirm that strength training is important in keeping functional age low. Indeed, its benefits become even more crucial as you grow older.

If you are part of the largest group of seniors, those who have noticed a marked decrease in their strength, flexibility, and balance, but who still function more or less independently, then clearly, it's time to dust off those weights and get started! Here is how to work, and what to watch for, in order to bring back the strength you have lost.

■ **Obtain clearance from your doctor first.** If you are sedentary and over 65, you should have a cardiac stress test before starting to exercise. Your doctor may also advise a respiratory function test, and a bone density scan. These exams will help you feel more confident and also provide a bottom-line medical record, one you will enjoy watching improve as you grow fitter.

■ **Warm up for at least 10–15 minutes before exercising.** Gentle, rhythmic movements, such as easy leg and arm swings, shoulder circles, arm reaches, and ankle circles make a good warm-up. A brisk walk, dancing, or even marching in place will also suffice. Remember, your aim is to increase your circulation and the depth of your breathing, but you should still be able to speak easily. (See also page 21.)

■ **Cool down at the end of your workout.** Stopping too abruptly after a vigorous workout will strain your heart. Five to 10 minutes of slow, gentle stretching will give your pulse a chance to return to normal.

■ **Never, ever, ever hold your breath!** Especially, be sure not to hold your breath when doing an exertive movement such as lifting a weight. Exhale on the hardest part of the exercise (usually the lift), and inhale on the recovery.

■ **At first, do the exercises without using weights.** Once you have learned the correct form and are sure you are breathing correctly, you may begin to use light weights. As your strength builds, increase the number of repetitions. After about 4–6 weeks you can begin to add weight, but only in small increments—just a pound or two at the most. Stick with this for at least 4 weeks before deciding if you need to go higher.

■ **Trust your instincts. Don't strain, or do anything that hurts, or intimidates you.** You are the expert in your own body, and know best how to pace yourself. But if you are not meeting your fitness goals, or cannot motivate yourself, consider hiring a personal trainer, or join a group class. Make sure the instructor is well qualified and has experience working with seniors.

■ **Be constantly aware of correct alignment.** Before doing any movement, take a minute and check to be sure that your abdominal core is active, your chest is open and lifted, and your lower back is in a safe, neutral curve.

■ **Do not rush any exercises, or use momentum** when lifting or lowering weights.

■ **Be extremely cautious when doing any stretches or movements involving the neck.** You may simply choose to eliminate these actions, and should do so if you know you have arthritis in the neck.

■ **Keep your hands and fingers strong and flexible.** Squeeze a tennis ball. Pretend to play the piano. Hold your hands in soft fists, and then rotate them at the wrists. Press your palms together as if you are saying your prayers, and lift the elbows to the sides; notice the stretch this creates.

■ **Practice balance every day.** Not only will you reduce your chances of falling, but the exercises themselves build strength in the hips, legs, ankles, and feet.

■ **Be consistent in your exercise practice.** It is generally accepted that in order to build strength, you need to work out at least three times a week, taking a day or two to rest in between. Some people prefer to exercise daily, working different muscle groups each day in order to avoid overdoing it. A little exercise every day is infinitely better than a once-weekly binge.

■ **Commit to the exercise habit,** the same way you are committed to brushing your teeth. By exercising at least 3 times a week, it will soon become a habit. This is very important in determining your ongoing success. In time you will notice that you always feel better after exercising.

It may even become something you look forward to! At that point, your motivation is assured, and you will have achieved an important victory over premature aging.

■ **Try not to compare yourself to others.** Everyone's body and mind ages differently. So what if that old guy down the block walks faster than you do? Compete with no one, especially not your younger self. Stay focussed on the fact that by committing to exercise you are doing yourself and your family a big, loving favor. Congratulate yourself for having the courage to try something new. Celebrate the fact that you have taken a step toward managing your own well-being, and a step away from dependence on doctors and medication. Enjoy how exercise makes you feel. The fact that you have decided to exercise is a tremendous accomplishment, and one you can be proud of!

Here are some important strengthening exercises for everyone to do on a regular basis

■ Flat Belly Exhale (page 23)
■ Heel Slide (page 24)
■ Table 1 (pages 108–109)
■ Table 2 (page 110)
■ Oblique Curl-Up (if you do not have osteoporosis) (page 111)
■ Scapular Squeeze (page 31)
■ The Bridge (page 103)
■ Squats (pages 37–41)—modify if necessary)
■ Ankle Flex against Resistance (page 80)
■ Heel Raises (page 78)
■ Balance Exercises (pages 124–127)

Chair Exercises for Strength

Even if you cannot get down on the floor or stand without a cane or walker, you can still build strength. Most standing exercises, especially those that build arm and shoulder strength, can also be done seated on a chair. Be sure the seat of the chair is firm and level, and that the back is straight. The alignment rule of ear-above-shoulder-above hip still applies. When seated, maintain the natural (forward) curve of your lower back (page 107). Place a pillow behind you if, in spite of your best intentions, you find your lower spine sinks backward against the chair.

Here are a few exercises you can do in your chair

- Kegels (page 26)
- Scapular Squeeze (page 31)
- Up against the Wall (page 35)
- Biceps Curl (page 94)
- Kickbacks, Standing (page 96)
- Front Raise, Standing (page 85)
- Lateral Raise (page 92)
- Ankle Flex against Resistance (page 80)
- Heel Raises (page 78: sit on a chair and raise your heels. Put a dumbbell on each thigh for more challenge).

Squats are an excellent exercise to do to build strength in the lower body, but you might want to modify them as follows: Stand in front of a stable chair with your arms crossed in front of your chest and your legs slightly wider than hip-width apart. Slowly bend your knees and hinge your hips backward until you are seated. Then, keeping your back straight, lean forward and reverse the action to stand back up. Do this 10 times, then rest. Repeat the set if you can. (If this is too strenuous, don't lower your bottom all the way down to the chair before you stand back up.)

Floor Exercises—Without Getting Down on the Floor!

If getting down onto the floor is difficult for you, here is an easy adaptation to make: All of the lower body exercises done in a prone (face down), supine (face up), or side-lying position can be done on a firm bed. A wooden bedboard, or even an old door slipped under your mattress, will help create a hard-enough surface to provide adequate support and resistance.

Chair Exercises for Flexibility

These stretches are almost as effective done in a chair as on the floor. The only thing left out is the lower back stretch that occurs when you lie on your back. Note: These are excellent stretches for anyone to do to keep from getting stiff during long rides, or when stuck at a desk.

Seated Cat/Cow   level: beginning

benefits: Stretches the upper and lower back, as well as the chest muscles. Encourages deep breathing, relaxation, and stress reduction.

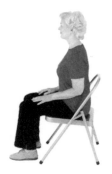

1 Sit toward the front edge of a stable chair, with your feet flat on the floor. Your legs should be hip-width apart and parallel to each other. Be sure you are seated in good alignment, balanced on the two "sit bones" (page 107) and maintaining your spine's natural curves. Rest your palms on top of your thighs.

2 Inhale deeply and fully, as you lift and arch your chest forward. Feel as if your chest is filled with helium, and is floating upward. Your focus will rise slightly, but keep your neck long and don't allow the head to fall backward. Squeeze the shoulder blades in toward each other to support the arch. This is the "cow."

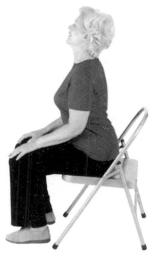

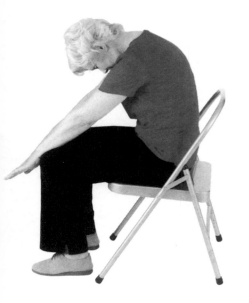

3 Exhale, and roll toward the back of your sit-bones. Pull the abdominal muscles in and up, and allow the chin to tuck into the chest. Your lower back will round toward the back of the chair, and you will feel a good stretch along the length and width of your back. This is the "cat."

4 Repeat at least four more times. Always coordinate the breath with the action.

Seated Crossover Stretch   level: beginning

benefits: Great for anyone who sits for long periods of time.

tips: If this causes pain in the crossed knee, try flexing that foot. If it still hurts, then this stretch is not a beneficial one for you at this time.

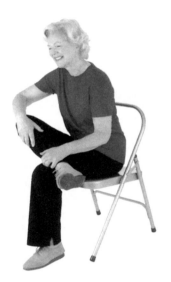

1 Sit as for Step 1, page 133, then place the outside of your right ankle on top of your left thigh, near the knee. (Use your hands to place the ankle in position, if necessary.)

2 Still sitting tall, hinge forward from the hips until you feel a stretch in the right hip area. You may not need to move much at all for this to occur! Hold this stretch for 4–6 breaths, then return the right foot to the floor. Repeat on the other side.

Seated Spiral Stretch   level: beginning

benefits: Stretches the shoulders, upper and lower back muscles, and lengthens the spine. Encourages relaxation.

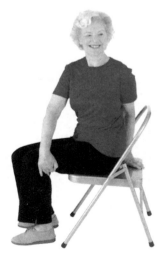

1 Sit as for Step 1, page 133, then stretch your rib cage up and turn your shoulders to the left, until you feel a stretch. Push your right hand gently against the outside of your left thigh and hold the chair with your left hand for support. Keep the chest lifted, and relax the shoulders. Breathe deeply and fully for 4–6 breaths.

2 Unwind to return to the front, rest for a moment, then repeat to the other side.

Seated Hamstring Stretch   level: beginning

benefits: Stretches the strong muscles on the back of the thighs. This may help relieve lower back tightness, too.

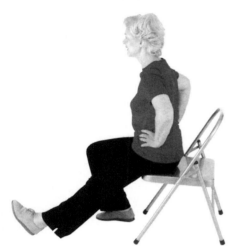

1 Sit as for Step 1, page 133, then place the heel of your left foot on the floor in front of your left hip, straightening that knee.

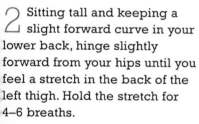

2 Sitting tall and keeping a slight forward curve in your lower back, hinge slightly forward from your hips until you feel a stretch in the back of the left thigh. Hold the stretch for 4–6 breaths.

3 Repeat on the other side.

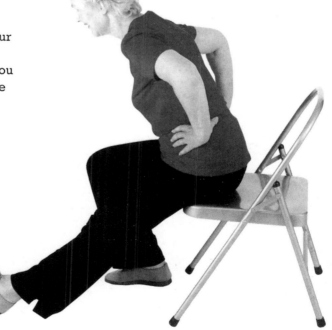

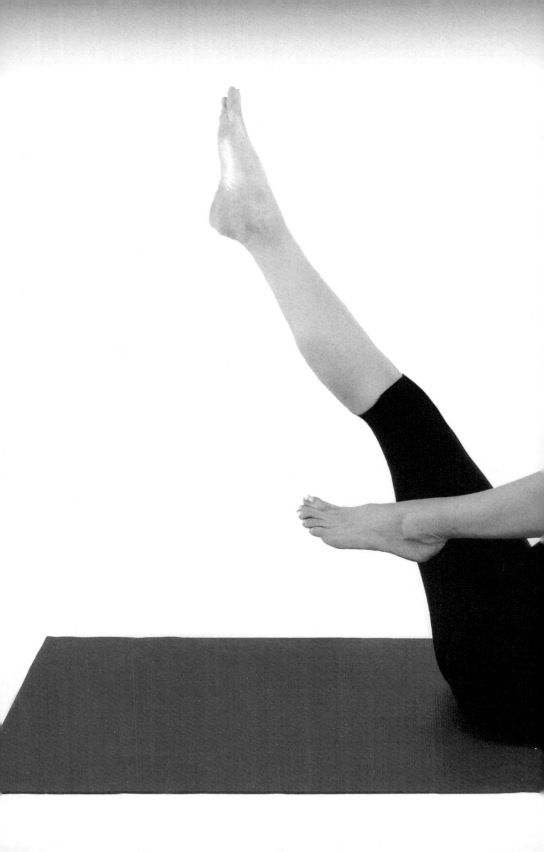

part 4 the programs

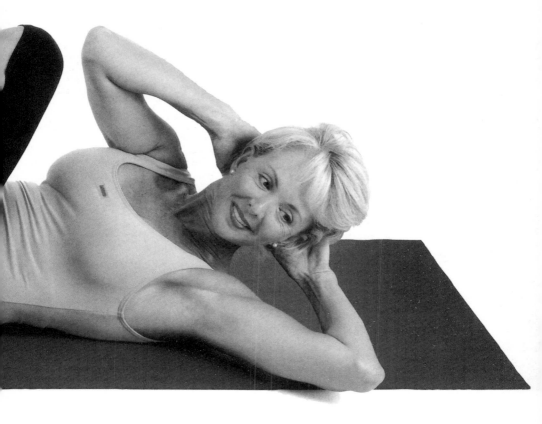

Beginning Workout 1:
Lower Body and Back

If you have never worked out at all, this is a safe and effective start for strength building. It's also a good reintroduction if you've been away from exercise for a while. Commit to exercising at least three times a week, alternating between Beginning

Workout 1 one day, and Beginning Workout 2 the next. Practice the Flat Belly Exhale (pages 23) and Kegels (page 26) daily and don't forget to warm up for at least 10 minutes before you start. Form is more important than speed or number of reps.

Core, Foundation, and Balance

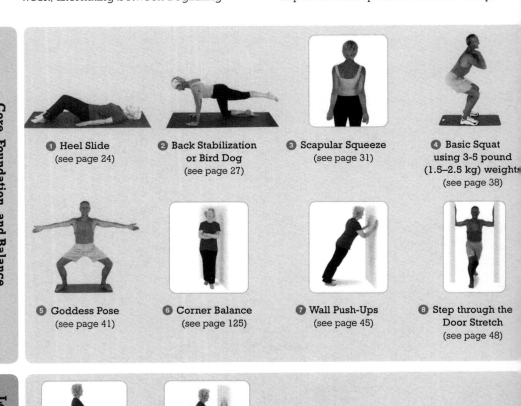

❶ **Heel Slide**
(see page 24)

❷ **Back Stabilization or Bird Dog**
(see page 27)

❸ **Scapular Squeeze**
(see page 31)

❹ **Basic Squat using 3-5 pound (1.5–2.5 kg) weights**
(see page 38)

❺ **Goddess Pose**
(see page 41)

❻ **Corner Balance**
(see page 125)

❼ **Wall Push-Ups**
(see page 45)

❽ **Step through the Door Stretch**
(see page 48)

Lower Body and Back

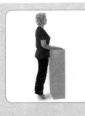

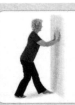

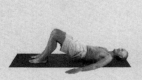

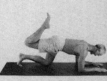

❾ **Heel Raises**
(see page 78)

❿ **Gastrocnemius Stretch**
(see page 79)

⓫ **Tail Tucks**
(see page 53)

⓬ **Hamstring Curls**
(see page 56)

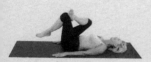

13 Crossover Stretch
(see page 42)

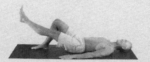

14 Supine Leg Lift
(see page 61)

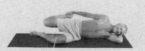

15 Quads Stretch
(see page 62)

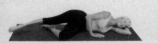

16 Side-Lying Leg Lifts
for Abductors
(see page 70)

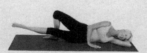

17 Side-Lying Leg Lifts
for Adductors
(see page 64)

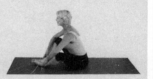

18 The Potted Plant Stretch
(see page 68)

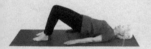

19 The Bridge
(see page 103)

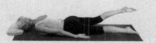

20 Half-Locust
(see page 104)

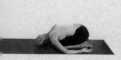

21 Child's Pose
(see page 28)

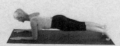

22 The Plank
(see page 117)

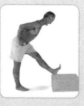

23 Standing
Hamstrings Stretch
(see page 58)

24 Legs up the
Wall Pose
(see page 120)

Lower Body and Back (cont.)

Putting it all Together,
Stretches, and Cool-Down

Beginning Workout 2:
Upper Body and Abdominals

When strengthening the upper body muscles, it is important to keep your lower back in good alignment. If not, your back may arch and strain as you lift the heavier weights. Remember always to engage the deep, lower core muscles of the abdomen, even while doing seemingly unrelated actions, such as the bicep curls or the Woodchopper. This is the essence of working from the "inside, out." By doing so, every exercise you perform, no matter how specific, will benefit your entire body.

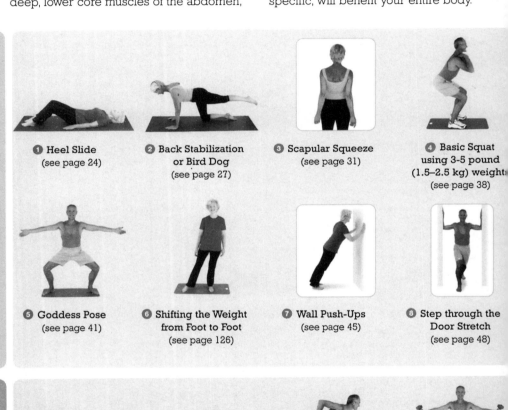

❶ Heel Slide
(see page 24)

❷ Back Stabilization or Bird Dog
(see page 27)

❸ Scapular Squeeze
(see page 31)

❹ Basic Squat using 3-5 pound (1.5–2.5 kg) weights
(see page 38)

❺ Goddess Pose
(see page 41)

❻ Shifting the Weight from Foot to Foot
(see page 126)

❼ Wall Push-Ups
(see page 45)

❽ Step through the Door Stretch
(see page 48)

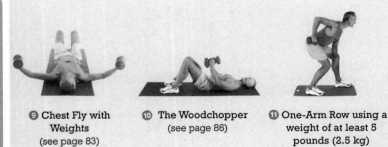
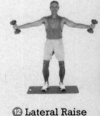

❾ Chest Fly with Weights
(see page 83)

❿ The Woodchopper
(see page 86)

⓫ One-Arm Row using a weight of at least 5 pounds (2.5 kg)
(see page 90)

⓬ Lateral Raise
(see page 92)

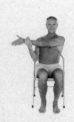

13 Pull-Across Stretch
for Shoulders
(see page 91)

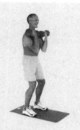

14 Biceps Curl using
weights of at least 5 pounds
(2.5 kg)
(see page 94)

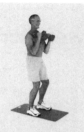

15 Hammer Curl
(see page 95)

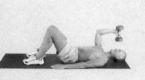

16 Triceps Extensions, Supine
(see page 97)

17 Scratch Your Back Stretch
(see page 99)

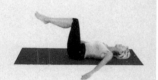

18 Table 1
(see page 108)

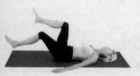

19 Table 2
(see page 110)

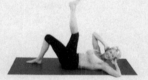

20 Oblique Curl-Up
(see page 111)

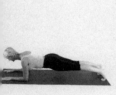

21 The Plank
(see page 117)

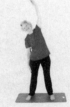

22 Standing Side Stretch
(see page 113)

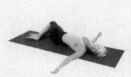

23 Spiral Stretch
(see page 76)

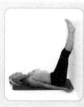

24 Legs up the
Wall Pose
(see page 120)

Intermediate–Advanced Workout 1: Lower Body and Back

At this point, you should be ready to slightly increase the weight of your dumbbells. Continue to "tune in" to your body's signals; use them to decide when to progress to more difficult variations, or do another set of reps. As your muscles grow stronger, they will augment each other's work. Suddenly you notice that what used to be difficult now feels easy, even pleasant! Your muscles will become more defined, and you will feel your energy growing steadily, and lasting longer.

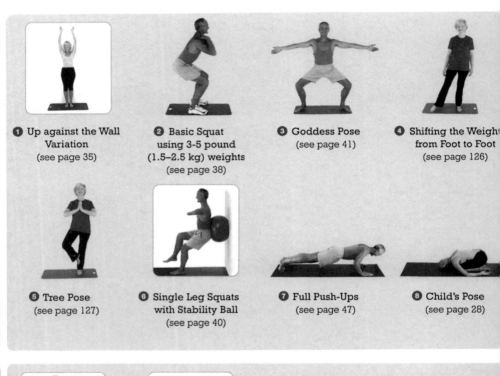

1 Up against the Wall Variation (see page 35)

2 Basic Squat using 3-5 pound (1.5–2.5 kg) weights (see page 38)

3 Goddess Pose (see page 41)

4 Shifting the Weight from Foot to Foot (see page 126)

5 Tree Pose (see page 127)

6 Single Leg Squats with Stability Ball (see page 40)

7 Full Push-Ups (see page 47)

8 Child's Pose (see page 28)

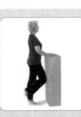
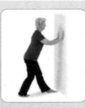
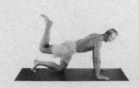
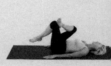

9 Heel Raises Variation 1 (see page 78)

10 Gastrocnemius Stretch (see page 79)

11 Butt Lifter (see page 54)

12 Crossover Stretch (see page 42)

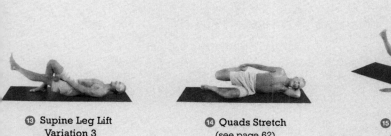
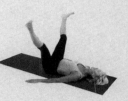

13 Supine Leg Lift
Variation 3
(see page 61)

14 Quads Stretch
(see page 62)

15 The Scissors
(see page 66)

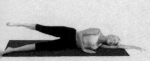
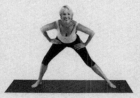
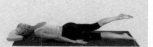

16 Front and Back Swing
(see page 74)

17 Standing Adductor
Stretch with Plié
(see page 69)

18 Half-Locust
(see page 104)

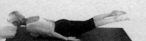
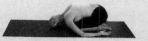

19 The Boat
(see page 105)

20 Child's Pose
(see page 28)

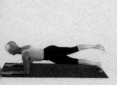
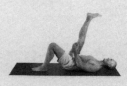
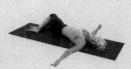
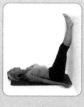

21 Plank with
Leg Raise
(see page 118)

22 Supine Hamstrings
Stretch
(see page 59)

23 Spiral Stretch
(see page 76)

24 Legs up the
Wall Pose
(see page 120)

Intermediate–Advanced Workout 2: Upper Body and Abdominals

Due to the overload principal, muscles grow strong in response to repeating the same actions over and over. At some point, however, the muscles become so efficient at performing it, the challenge ceases. Your progress may slow or even stall at this point. Avoid this by doing a new exercise or variation every few weeks. For example, do the push-ups with your hands closer together (or farther apart) than you usually do, and feel how differently the muscles respond.

Foundational and Balance

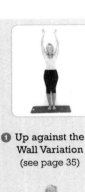

1 Up against the Wall Variation (see page 35)

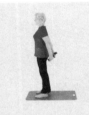

2 Scapular Squeeze with weights (see page 32)

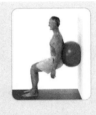

3 Squats with Stability Ball Variation (see page 39)

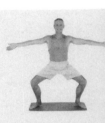

4 Goddess Pose (see page 41)

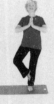

5 Tree Pose (see page 127)

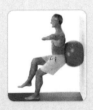

6 Single Leg Squats with Stability Ball, but holding weights (see page 40)

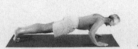

7 Full Push-Ups (see page 47)

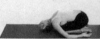

8 Child's Pose (see page 28)

Upper Body and Abdominals

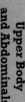

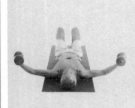

9 Chest Fly with Weights (see page 83)

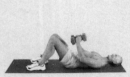

10 The Woodchopper (see page 86)

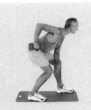

11 One Arm Row using a heavier weight (see page 90)

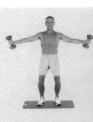

12 Lateral Raise (see page 92)

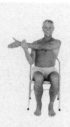

13 Pull-Across Stretch for Shoulders
(see page 91)

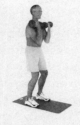

14 Biceps Curl using weights of at least 5 pounds (2.5 kg)
(see page 94)

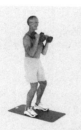

15 Hammer Curl using weights of at least 5 pounds (2.5 kg)
(see page 95)

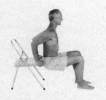

16 Triceps Dips
(see page 98)

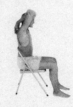

17 Scratch Your Back Stretch
(see page 99)

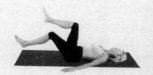

18 Table 2
(see page 110)

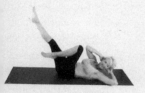

19 Bicycle Crunch
(see page 112)

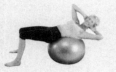

20 Stability Ball Curl-Up
(see page 114)

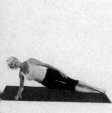

21 Side-Lying Plank
(see page 119)

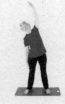

22 Standing Side Stretch
(see page 113)

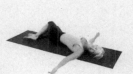

23 Spiral Stretch
(see page 76)

24 Legs up the Wall Pose
(see page 120)

Fifteen-Minute Workout

There is no need to miss your workout just because you are pressed for time. Here is a way to exercise the major muscle groups necessary for general fitness, while still leaving time to target a specific muscle group or two, and even finish with a couple of stretches. This program is for an average, intermediate-level adult. If you like, you can do exercises of your choice during the last five minutes. As long as you always warm up, do Squats and Push-Ups first, and finish with stretches (which double as a cool-down), you will have done a safe and well-rounded workout.

First 5 minutes

Do your warm-up. Go for a brisk walk, ride a bike, climb a few flights of stairs, dance to your favorite CD...whatever you choose, be sure it is vigorous enough to raise your heart rate, increase the depth of your breathing, and stir your blood into circulation.

Next 5 minutes

❶ Do one set of 10–15 Squats. Choose a variation appropriate to your fitness level; here we show the Door Squat.

❷ Follow with a set of 10 Push-Ups of your choice; here it is Knee Push-Ups.

❸ Do another set of 10–15 Squats, progressing to a more challenging level, if you'd like.

❹ Follow with another set of 10 Push-Ups. Remember to select a variation that challenges you enough that it is difficult, and yet you can maintain correct form.

❺ and ❻ Repeat, alternating one set of Squats, (either the ones you did previously or a different variation), with one set of challenging enough Push-Ups. By now, your upper and lower body should feel as if they have worked.

❼ Next, do a set of 20 Bicycle Crunches.

❽ Alternate this with the Bridge, holding it for 4 breaths, and lowering your spine slowly back down to the floor.

❾ and ❿ Repeat the set of 20 Bicycle Crunches, followed by another Bridge.

Last 5 minutes

❿ or ⓫ Strengthen your back with the Half-Locust (6 times, alternating legs), followed by either another repetition of the same, or the Boat (hold for 4 breaths, lower and rest, and repeat twice more).

⓭ Roll onto your back, and do the Rock and Roll Stretch.

⓮ or ⓯ Follow with a Supine Hamstring Stretch or a Spiral Stretch. Roll onto your side to stand up. Inhale deeply as you raise your arms overhead, reaching up until you feel a good stretch in your entire body. Exhale and slowly lower the arms. You're done!

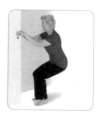

❶ Door Squat
(see page 37)

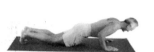

❷ Knee Push-Ups
(see page 46)

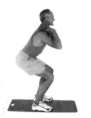

❸ Basic Squat
(see page 38)

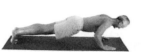

❹ Full Push-Ups
(see page 47)

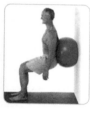

❺ Squats with Stability Ball
(see page 39)

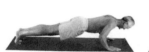

❻ Full Push-Ups
(see page 47)

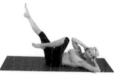

❼ Bicycle Crunch
(see page 112)

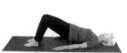

❽ The Bridge
(see page 103)

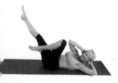

❾ Bicycle Crunch
(see page 112)

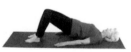

❿ The Bridge
(see page 103)

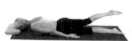

⓫ Half-Locust
(see page 104)

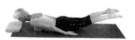

⓬ The Boat
(see page 105)

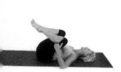

Rock and Roll Stretch
(see page 29)

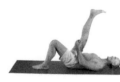

⓮ Supine Hamstrings Stretch
(see page 59)

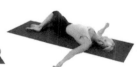

⓯ Spiral Stretch
(see page 76)

On the Road Workout

Travel can exact a heavy price on your fitness. But it doesn't have to be that way. Here is how you can fit strength and flexibility exercises into your schedule, even if your hotel doesn't have a four-star gym.

On the plane/train

❶ Be certain that you are seated with your back in its neutral, or "strong back curve" (page 107). Place a rolled-up blanket, or purse, or sweater behind your lower back to support it. Now strengthen your core muscles. Do the Kegels exercise (see page 26), and pull your deep abdominal muscles in and up.

Are your shoulders tense? Circle them up, back, and down a few times, and take deep "belly breaths" (see page 19).

❷ Now do Scapular Squeezes. They help realign your upper body and make it easier to relax your shoulders and neck.

❸ The Scratch Your Back Stretch will keep the circulation flowing in your upper body and feels great, too.

❹ Now stretch your back by doing the Seated Cat/Cow.

❺ Follow this with the Seated Spiral Stretch. (This one has the additional advantage of not looking too conspicuous!)

❻ and ❼ Bring circulation into your ankles by doing Ankle Flex against Resistance and the Foot Point Stretch. This will help keep any swelling down, and may even prevent dangerous embolisms from forming.

❽ Stretch out tight hip and lower back muscles with the Seated Crossover Stretch. Remember, however, not to push these stretches since you won't be warmed up. The purpose here is just to get your circulation going.

At your hotel

❾ After a 10-minute warm-up of your choice (you could climb several flights of stairs) do as many Up against the Wall Variations as required, to stretch out tense shoulder and back muscles.

❿ and ⓫ Do three sets of Basic Squats alternating with three sets of Wall Push-Ups.

⓬ Work your abdominals by doing two or three sets of Bicycle Crunches.

⓭ Strengthen your back with Half-Locust.

⓮ Relax and stretch your legs and back with Standing Hamstrings Stretches.

⓯ Continue to unwind with the Spiral Stretch.

⓰ Finish with Legs up the Wall Pose. This is especially good after a day in and out of airports, as it helps reduce the swelling in your legs and feet.

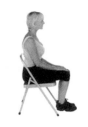

1 Correct Sitting
(see page 107)

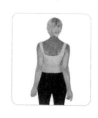

2 Scapular Squeeze
(see page 31)

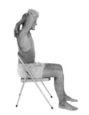

3 Scratch Your
Back Stretch
(see page 99)

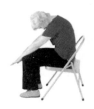

4 Seated Cat/Cow
(see page 133)

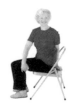

5 Seated Spiral
Stretch
(see page 134)

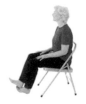

6 Ankle Flex against
Resistance
(see page 80)

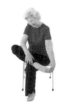

7 Foot Point Stretch
(see page 81)

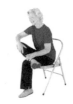

8 Seated Crossover
Stretch
(see page 134)

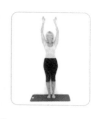

9 Up against the Wall
Variation
(see page 35)

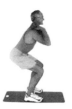

10 Basic Squat
(see page 38)

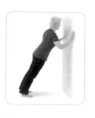

11 Wall Push-Up
(see page 45)

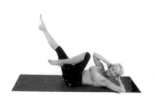

12 Bicycle Crunch
(see page 112)

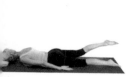

13 Half-Locust
(see page 104)

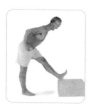

14 Standing
Hamstrings Stretch
(see page 58)

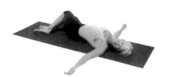

15 Spiral Stretch
(see page 76)

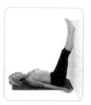

16 Legs up the
Wall Pose
(see page 120)

Lower Back Workout

It is a rare over-50-year-old who has never experienced low back pain. (Studies estimate back pain is responsible for 80 percent of job absenteeism.) The first thing to do is evaluate your posture (see pages 18–19). Chances are high that your pain is emanating, at least in part, from faulty alignment. Improve your alignment by strengthening your lower core.

Be sure to check with your doctor before doing any of the following exercises. If you have no injury or condition that precludes exercise, then do them daily until you get relief.

❶,❷, and ❸ Do the Flat Belly Exhale, the Heel Slide and the Kegels exercise (see page 26), as well as the Back Stabilization Exercise daily, or even twice a day.

❹ and ❺ Follow with the Rock and Roll Stretch and Child's Pose to gently stretch tight lower back muscles.

❻ Usually the upper body is also out of alignment when the lower back is weak. Remedy this by doing lots of Scapular Squeezes! This will help to bring your head into correct alignment above your spine, which will also bring relief to your lower back.

❼ The Cat/Cow will serve as both a stretch and a mild strengthener. Coordinate your breath with the movements for best results. Do the Cat/Cow as many times as you need, until you begin to feel a sense of fluidity and length in your entire spine, directing the stretch to the places where you "need it" the most.

❽ Strengthen your back further with the Half-Locust. Keep the leg low. Pull your abdominal muscles in and up the entire time. Think of this as a breathing exercise; that way, you will avoid additional stress on your back muscles.

❾ Afterward, rest and stretch in Child's Pose.

❿ or ⓫, and ⓬, or ❿ or ⓫ and ⓭ Good abdominal tone, especially in the oblique muscles, will help support your back. Do one or two sets of Table 1 or Table 2 and the Oblique Curl-Up. (If you have osteoporosis, skip the Oblique Curl-Ups and do Heel Slide instead.)

⓮ Follow your abdominal exercises with the The Bridge. Like the Cat/Cow, this will both strengthen and stretch your spine. Raise your hips only as high as it feels good.

⓯ A final factor to consider: How flexible are your hamstrings? Often, stretching those will take some of the strain off your lower back by allowing the pelvis to be positioned in correct alignment. Do the Supine Hamstrings Stretch in the slowest, gentlest way possible.

⓰ End with Legs up the Wall Pose.

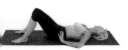

1 Flat Belly Exhale
(see page 23)

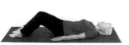

2 Heel Slide
(see page 24)

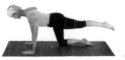

3 Back Stabilization
or Bird Dog
(see page 27)

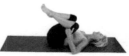

4 Rock and Roll
Stretch
(see page 29)

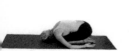

5 Child's Pose
(see page 28)

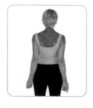

6 Scapular Squeeze
(see page 31)

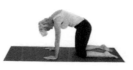

7 Cat/Cow Stretch
(see page 33)

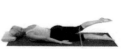

8 Half-Locust
(see page 104)

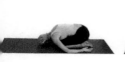

9 Child's Pose
(see page 28)

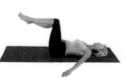

10 Table 1
(see page 108)

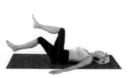

11 Table 2
(see page 110)

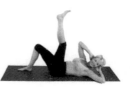

12 Oblique Curl-Up
(see page 111)

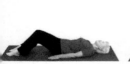

13 Heel Slide
(see page 24)

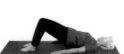

14 The Bridge
(see page 103)

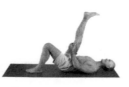

15 Supine Hamstrings
Stretch
(see page 59)

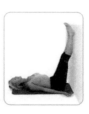

16 Legs up the
Wall Pose
(see page 120)

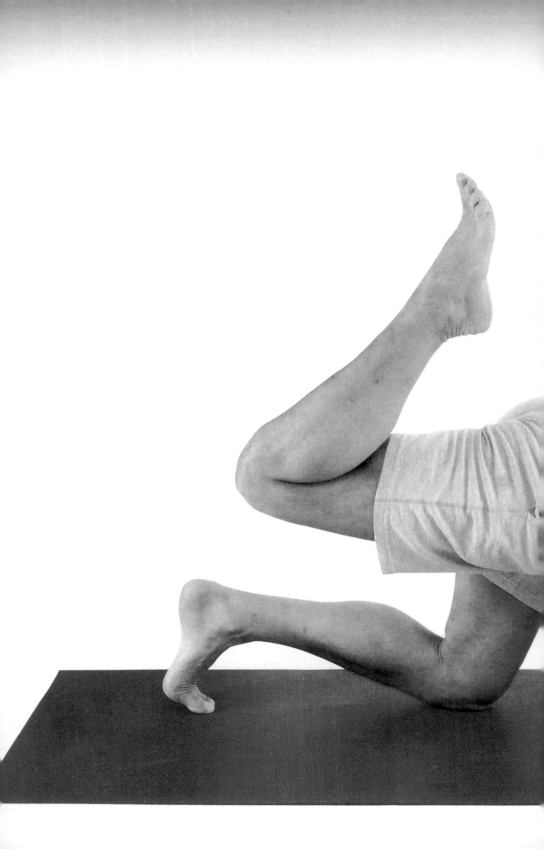

part 5 **appendix**

> **some basic nutritional guidelines for the over-50 exerciser**

> **sore muscles**

> **alternative forms of exercise**

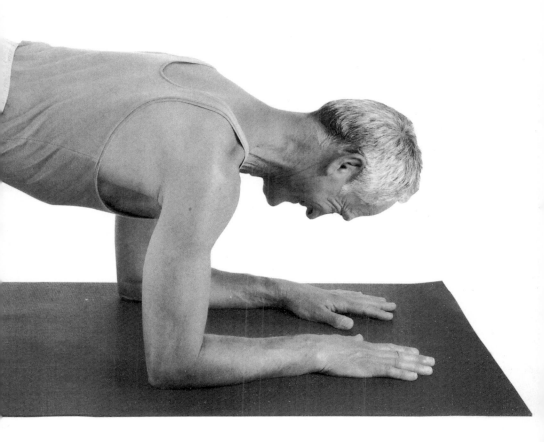

Some Basic Nutritional Guidelines for the Over-50 Exerciser

Nutritional advice is often complicated and even self-contradictory; no wonder it's hard to separate fact from fiction. The following simple nutritional strategies, all based on solid research, may enhance your health, energy, and ability to build strength.

First, make sure that about 60 percent of your daily calorie intake comes from carbohydrates, no more than 30 percent comes from fat, and between 10 percent and 20 percent comes from protein. This translates into lots of carbohydrates, moderate amounts of protein, and small amounts of fat.

Carbohydrates supply energy. Nutritionally valuable complex carbohydrates such as fruits, vegetables, whole-grained products, and legumes, provide multitudes of vitamins, minerals, and disease-fighting phytochemicals as well as fiber. Try to eat 8 to 10 servings of fruit and vegetables a day, especially the brightly colored ones that pack the most nutritional value. The empty calories in refined carbohydrates such as candy, cookies, and white bread will only increase your weight and make you even hungrier later.(Alcohol falls into this category, too.)

We need a certain amount of fat in our diet, but the kind you choose is as important as the quantity. Avocados, nuts, and coldwater fish such as salmon and sardines all contain oils and fatty acids that are very good for you, especially your heart. Cook with healthy monosaturated oils such as olive and canola. Saturated fats, found in dairy products and meats, should be severely limited; select low-fat cheeses, milk, and yogurt—that way you won't miss out on the important calcium they supply. Avoid artery-clogging polyunsaturated or trans fats that lurk in baked and processed foods. (The label will say "hydrogenated" or "partially hydrogenated.")

Protein is essential for building muscle. An inadequate intake may contribute to sarcopenia (page 10) in older adults. Fish, skinless chicken, soy, low-fat dairy, egg whites, and lean cuts of meat are all good sources. Because it is digested slowly and steadily, include some high-quality protein in every meal; it helps sustain your energy level throughout the day. Note: High-protein, low-carbohydrate diets are not a magic bullet for sustainable weight loss, and can lead to serious health problems.

Nutritional Supplements

The best way to get the vitamins, minerals, and other trace elements you need is by eating a wide variety of fresh, unprocessed foods. A good multivitamin may be adequate to fill in the missing pieces of an imperfect diet. But some very interesting research has begun to reveal that certain vitamins and minerals have even more health-promoting properties than was previously realized, especially for those over age 50. These antioxidants as they are called, guard against disease, strengthen the immune system, and even slow aging. They accomplish this by neutralizing free-radicals, the natural by-products of metabolism that can lead to cellular damage. Here are a few supplements to consider (check with your health-care professional for the correct recommended amounts).

Vitamin C

Humans don't produce their own vitamin C, so you need to replace this water-soluble vitamin every day. Along with vitamins A, B-6, E, and the minerals copper, iron, selenium, and zinc, it has important immunity-boosting and disease-preventive properties. It also helps to build collagen and increases iron absorption.

Vitamin E

Vitamin E may reduce the risk of cancer, cardiovascular disease, and even Alzheimer's disease. It is a powerful antioxidant, but chances are you are getting enough if you include nuts, vegetable oil, and leafy greens in your diet. Avoid overdoing it: you need no more than 150 IU, the amount typically provided by a multivitamin. Large amounts (more than 1000 IU) raise the risk of internal bleeding.

Vitamin B-12

Because of reduced stomach acid, up to one-third of people over 50 can't synthesize this vitamin, found in meat, dairy, poultry, and fish. It reduces the amount of homocysteine in the blood, an amino acid that at elevated levels contributes to arteriosclerosis, heart disease, and stroke. (If you are a vegetarian, it is definitely recommended that you supplement with vitamin B-12.)

Calcium and Vitamin D

Along with exercise, an adequate calcium supply is indispensable for strong bones. This applies to men over 60 as well as to all women. Calcium supports nerve and muscle function and prevents high blood pressure, too. You can get calcium from dairy products, fortified orange juice, and sardines. Most Americans get only about half the recommended daily supply of calcium from their diet, however. That's why it's wise to supplement with up to 1,500 mg of calcium a day. Choose a supplement containing vitamin D; recent studies conclude this vitamin is more important than previously thought for maintaining healthy bones.

Water

It is always important to drink enough water but especially so when you exercise. It cools the body, circulates blood to the muscles and organs, and lubricates all the joints. Dehydration reduces the volume of your blood, making it thick, sluggish, and unable to provide sufficient oxygen to the brain to keep you thinking clearly. That is why you may sometimes feel groggy and fatigued on hot, humid days or after you have done a long hard workout.

Even a little dehydration can cause big problems. These include elevated heart rate, electrolyte imbalance, and dizziness. The American College of Sports Medicine recommends drinking a glass or two of water before exercising, to give your body time to adjust its fluid levels. Replenish your water supply throughout your workout; the body can lose as much as 3 pints (1.5 liters) of fluid in an hour of moderate exercise.

You also need to be warned that the body is notoriously poor at registering thirst. This inability to sense thirst worsens as you age, when your ability to conserve water is already diminished, due to changes in kidney function. Drink water (or noncaffeinated, nonalcoholic, nonsugary beverages) often. Drink more than you believe you need, and you'll be fine. You may even notice a marked improvement in your exercise performance and your energy levels.

Sore Muscles

Building strength is a dance between pushing your muscles beyond their usual performance and then resting to allow them time to repair and grow stronger. Sometimes, a day or so after pushing them a bit too hard, your muscles may feel stiff and sore. You haven't strained them, exactly, but the discomfort is severe enough that it interferes with your ability to exercise for the next few days. Researchers call this exercise-induced soreness Delayed Onset Muscle Soreness (DOMS) and have focused on identifying why it occurs and how to prevent it.

You may have heard that muscle soreness results when lactic acid builds up in the muscle. This has been disproved. Instead, it appears that overdoing actions that emphasize eccentric contraction leads to DOMS. Briefly, muscles contract in several ways. They can shorten toward their center, as when you lift a dumbbell in a biceps curl. They can maintain their length as they work; this is called isometric contraction. In eccentric contraction, the muscle lengthens as it contracts, giving you the power to lower a heavy weight slowly and with control, or to sit back into a deep squat without falling on your bottom. Indeed it is during the eccentric phase of a movement (that is, the lowering of the dumbbell rather than the lifting of it) that the most strengthening has been proven to take place.

Clearly, the challenge is to learn how to do strengthening, eccentric contractions without ending up with a bad case of sore muscles. Happily, this is easy to do, and here's how:

❶ Always warm up first before strength training. The more out of shape you are, the longer your warm-up should be. Do a general warm-up of anywhere from 10 to 20 minutes to raise your body's temperature. Follow this with a specific warm-up focusing on the actions you are about to perform. In other words, if you plan to work your leg muscles, be sure to include some gentle leg movements in your warm-up. (In this book the Squats serve this purpose.)

❷ When you are ready to increase the intensity of your workout, do so gradually and moderately. Increase the weight of your dumbbells by only a pound or two at a time. Add more repetitions over the course of weeks, not days.

❸ Know that as your muscles adapt over time to the work they are doing, the likelihood of getting sore will diminish.

What if, despite all your sensible precautions, you worked harder than you realized and now your muscles are really killing you? Common sense prevails. Rest. This is not the time to "Work through it." Hot baths sometimes help speed up the healing, and some doctors recommend antiinflammatory medication such as aspirin or ibuprofen, but the studies are mixed here. Once your muscle soreness has down-graded into stiffness, it's time to climb back in the saddle. (Just make sure that you warm up first.)

Alternative Forms of Exercise

You may want to explore some of these exercise forms to augment your strength training. Doing a variety of exercises will encourage your muscles to move in new and different ways. This is a good way to stay motivated, avoid burnout, and keep the muscles working at top form. Called cross-training in some circles, it is a smart move for the over-50s.

Yoga

There are good reasons why growing numbers of people are studying this ancient discipline. Yoga builds remarkable strength and flexibility. Its true power, however, lies in the way it leads you to tune in with clarity and acceptance to physical and emotional limitations, and then move beyond them. Yoga incorporates meditation and breath work, both of which have been proven to reduce stress, lower blood pressure, and enhance immunity. All of these factors make it a good choice for anyone, but especially for the over-50s.

Pilates

Wonderful for building core strength and for balancing toning with flexibility, this technique was developed by Joseph Pilates in the early 1900s while working with nonambulatory hospital patients. He attached springs to the patients' beds to help them move their limbs. Later, he created a series of spring-based exercise apparatuses to help students retrain the way they use their bodies. This equipment is still used, often by physical therapists. Most Pilates classes, however, are done lying on mats. You will learn how to stretch and strengthen your abdominals and back, and to use your core to stabilize alignment. (Sound familiar?)

Tai Chi and Qi Gong

Qi Gong (on which Tai Chi is based), was developed many centuries ago in China. Qi Gong practitioners believe that the body's energy ("Qi") flows in circular patterns, and they do specific movements to cultivate or strengthen this vital and health-promoting energy. The movements of Qi Gong are smooth and fluid, making it a great choice for those with arthritis. This gentle, meditative form of exercise is surprisingly strengthening for the cardiovascular system, lower body muscles, visual focus, and balance. Like Yoga, Qi Gong and Tai Chi bring the body, mind, and spirit into harmony, thus reducing stress.

Feldenkrais

Not a strength-building system per se, this method teaches you to move in a stress-free and efficient way. A highly trained Feldenkrais instructor will guide you through a series of subtle movements, specifically designed to retrain your neuromuscular system. This helps you let go of faulty, inefficient movement habits. Favored by professional athletes, dancers, musicians, and actors, Feldenkrais is recommended for both beginning and advanced exercisers, and is valuable in preventing and recovering from injury.

Index

A

abdominal muscles, 23, 102–15
  bicycle crunch, 112
  flat belly exhale, 23
  heel slide, 24–5
  oblique curl-up, 111
  the scissors, 66
  stability ball curl-up, 114–15
  supine leg lift, 61
  table, 108–10
  workouts, 140–1, 144–5
abductor muscles, 70
  balance, 124
  front and back swing, 74–5
  pizza circles, 72–3
  side-lying leg lift for
    abductors, 70–1
adductor muscles, 64
  the scissors, 66
  side-lying leg lift for
    adductors, 64–5
  standing adductor stretch
    with plié, 69
  wall sit with ball between
    the knees, 67
advanced workout, 142–5
aging
  functional age, 130
  loss of muscle mass, 10
  posture and, 18
alignment, 18–19, 130–1
ankle flex against resistance, 80
antioxidants, 154
arabesque with curls, 57
arm muscles see biceps
  muscles; deltoid muscles;
    triceps muscles
arthritis, 128–9

B

back, 27, 102–15
  arthritis, 129
  back stabilization
    (bird dog), 27
  the boat, 105
  the bridge, 103
  carrying technique, 107
  cat/cow stretch, 33
  child's pose, 28, 55
  half-locust, 104

lifting technique, 106
posture, 18
rock and roll stretch, 29
scapular squeeze, 31
scapular squeeze with
  weights, 32
up against the wall, 35
workouts, 138–9, 142–3, 150–1
balance, 124–7, 131
  corner balance, 125
  shifting the weight from
    foot to foot, 126
  tree pose, 127
balls see stability balls
beginning workout, 138–41
biceps muscles, 94
  biceps curl, 94
  hammer curl, 95
  "so big stretch", 95
bicycle crunch, 112
bird dog, 27
the boat, 105
bones
  alignment, 18–19, 130–1
  density, 10
  osteoporosis, 129
brain, stretch reflex, 17
breath, holding, 130
breathing, 16, 19, 120
the bridge, 103
butt lifter, 54
buttock muscles see
  gluteal muscles

C

calcium, 155
calf muscles see
  gastrocnemius muscles
calories, 10, 154
carbohydrates, 154
cardiac stress test, 130
cardiovascular system, 120–1
carrying technique, 107
cat/cow stretch, 33
  seated cat/cow, 133
"chain effect", 21
chair exercises, 132–5
  seated cat/cow, 133
  seated crossover stretch, 134
  seated hamstring stretch, 135
  seated spiral stretch, 134
chest muscles, 83
  chest fly with weights, 83

front raise, standing, 85
push-ups, 44–7
step through the door
  stretch, 48
supine chest stretch, 49,
  84, 115
child's pose, 28, 55
cooling-down, 120, 130
core support
  connecting upper and
    lower cores, 34
  lower body core, 22
  upper body core, 30
corner balance, 125
cow stretch, 33
  seated cow, 133
cramps, in toes, 81
crossover stretch, 42–3, 55, 75
  seated crossover stretch, 134
curl-ups
  oblique curl-up, 111
  stability ball curl-up, 114–15

D

deltoid muscles, 83, 88
  chest fly with weights, 83
  front raise, standing, 85
  lateral raise, 92
  one-arm row, 90
  reverse fly, 88–9
depression, 10
diabetes, 10
diet, 154–5
doctors, health checkups, 13, 130
door squat, 37
dorsi flexors (shin muscles), 14,
  52, 80, 124
  ankle flex against
    resistance, 80
drawbridge, 100–1

E

energy levels, 10
equipment, 12–13
erector spinae muscles, 103

F

falls, 80, 124
fat, in diet, 154
Feldenkrais, 157
fiber, 154
fifteen-minute workout, 146–7
fingers, flexibility, 131